The SECRET LIFE of a VET

The **SECRET LIFE** of a **VET**

RORY COWLAM

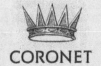

CORONET

First published in Great Britain in 2020 by Coronet
An Imprint of Hodder & Stoughton
An Hachette UK company

This paperback edition published in 2021

1

A CIP catalogue record for this title is available from the British Library

Paperback ISBN 9781529327847
eBook ISBN 9781529327823

Typeset in Adobe Garamond by Hewer Text UK Ltd, Edinburgh
Printed and bound in Great Britain by Clays Ltd, Elocraf S.p.A.

Hodder & Stoughton policy is to use papers that are natural, renewable
and recyclable products and made from wood grown in sustainable
forests. The logging and manufacturing processes are expected to
conform to the environmental regulations of the country of origin.

Hodder & Stoughton Ltd
Carmelite House
50 Victoria Embankment
London EC4Y 0DZ

www.hodder.co.uk

Firstly to my parents for always believing in me. Secondly, to the animals. It is a privilege to spend my life caring for you.

Contents

Introduction

I'm Rory.

I'm a companion animal vet working at The Neighbourhood Vet in South London. That essentially means I treat 'dogs and downwards', as I tell people when I meet them. I have had a passion for animals for as long as I can remember and as a child I was never without pets. From day one it seemed I had an affinity with animals. I was born into a house with cats, and they would often be found sitting near or next to me. It wasn't only the cats. As soon as I could crawl I was out in the garden exploring, collecting insects, fascinated by the natural world. Upon seeing that I was clearly a very young Dr Doolittle, my parents decided to get a dog when I was just four. They evidently knew I was going to be an animal lover, but not even they realised just to what extent.

I was a vet by the age of twenty-two, and having studied at one of the best veterinary schools in the world was now ready to become a practicing city vet. The veterinary profession is an incredible mish mash of high-tech medicine and surgery, and the beautiful innocence of caring for animals, and it all started for me at the tender age of four.

If you are reading this book thinking that being a veterinary professional is filled with cuddling cute puppies and kittens and giving a vaccination and a worming tablet, then I implore you to read on. It's so much more than that. Being a vet is an incredible career. I am privileged to be one and even more honoured to be able to give you a glimpse into it. My aim is to give you a sneaky peak into this ever-changing, topsy-turvy life. I want to cover it all: from a childhood fascinated with animals in the heart of the Cotswolds, through the insane world of veterinary school and into the early years of being a young vet fighting to stay afloat through blood, sweat and tears. It's all here. And, of course, it is all predictably but ever so rightly dedicated to the wonderful animals I am privileged enough to spend my life treating and helping in some small way.

1

In the Beginning

The first animal I shared a special connection with was a cat called Creamy. My mother adopted her before she had me, along with her sister Peaches, from the Cats Protection League. I loved Creamy and she loved me, sleeping next to me as a newborn baby and tucking herself in my pram while my mum wasn't looking.

People used to worry, having heard the horror stories of cats smothering babies in their cots, but I came to no harm and Creamy and I were inseparable. My parents loved to call her the 'guard cat' because she was always with me with one eye open to make sure I was okay. My mum told me stories as I got older about Creamy and her sister. My favourite was from 1988 in St Albans. Mum must have told me this a million times, and I used to recite it word for word when talking to whoever would listen to me about my love of animals. She told me how Creamy and Peaches were the most amazing cats, not a paw wrong until very early one morning she was woken by incessant meowing coming from outside. Now this was out of character – they were usually very independent cats – so she went downstairs and opened the front door.

Creamy was there on the front step, mewing and scratching at the door, carrying Peaches by the scruff. This amazing little black and white cat must have seen her sister stroll out into the road and take a glancing blow from a speeding car. She had picked her up and dragged her up the steep steps to the front door. Without her, Peaches wouldn't have survived. She was a true feline superhero.

By the time I was born, Peaches was no longer around. Creamy and her new adopted sister Topsy were the two animal residents of our home for the first three years of my life.

When I was four years old, however, my mum, my dad, my little sister and I went on a car journey that would change my life forever. We were off to pick up our first dog, Lulu. She was a blue Great Dane and she very quickly grew from the size of a rugby ball to twice the size of me. She instantly became my best friend and guardian. If you know the story of Peter Pan you will be familiar with my favourite character Nana (of course), the Darling family's dog. Lulu became my very own Nana, and would regularly look out for me when we were out and about. I used to ride my bicycle into school along with my sister Bethan, my mum and Lulu. We would cycle through the park and if I rode off too far ahead, Lulu was not far behind. If I ever got out of view of my mum, Lulu would grab onto my handlebars and not let go until my mum had caught up with us. It was bloody annoying, but what a dog! Back home, I quickly decided that wherever Lulu was, I needed to be. I would rush home from school and dive straight onto the floor by her bed, sitting there for hours on end. We played like siblings in the garden and shared a dog biscuit or two. She was my shadow and best friend. We have had many dogs over the years and I have loved every single one of them. But as I sit in my office writing now, though, there is a picture of Lulu on the bookshelf. We were kindred spirits.

*

I was born in Windsor but grew up in the Cotswolds, where I spent as much time around animals as possible. Despite being a fully fledged Londoner now, I still think of the Cotswolds as my spiritual home, with rolling fields filled with cows, sheep, pigs and horses, and windy backroads leading from farmstead to farmstead, bordered by hedges so high that you can only see over them from atop a tractor.

From the age of four until seven we lived in Cirencester in a tall townhouse with a long, thin garden. Lulu and I would run the length of the garden over and over and share an apple from the orchard. It was wonderful, but it wasn't until we moved out of the town to a little village called Hankerton that I felt like a proper country boy. The house sits nestled between three fields, with the nearest neighbour in a cottage at the end of the 200m driveway. My favourite part of the house was my 'forest', a wooded area at the back of the house with a huge horse chestnut tree at the centre. It was here that I spent a lot of my time with the dogs, collecting conkers, building bonfires and climbing trees. If I wasn't cuddling or playing with the dogs (after we got Lulu, it sort of opened the floodgates – we had three dogs for the majority of my childhood), I was out in the garden trying to learn as much as I could about nature. We had chickens and ducks and geese for a time, and – living surrounded by farmland – I was always off exploring. I was lucky to have parents who made sure to teach me as much about animals as possible, including involving me in raising and rearing animals for food production. And it wasn't uncommon for me to be helping my dad in the garden, growing enough vegetables to feed the village, or helping my mum in the kitchen where she passed on her love of cooking to me. Otherwise, in-between tormenting my little sister and playing with her in the garden, I was off finding insects or wildlife to learn about.

Our chickens and ducks provided the most amazing eggs, and it was my job to collect them in the morning before school as well as to fill up their food and water. At one point we had over a dozen hens and we had eggs coming out of our ears. I managed to persuade my mum that if I could sell the eggs and deliver them, I could keep the cash as pocket money. So off I went around the village on my bike, boxes of eggs stacked in a carrier bag swinging from my handlebars.

At weekends, I would help clean the chickens' enclosure out and bed them on clean straw. Ordinarily this was an easy job but then there was the cockerel. We had a number of cockerels over the years, and I thought they were wonderful, providing fertilised eggs for us to hatch into cute little chicks. Although a bit feisty they were manageable – then, for a few years there was Rocky Del Boy the Third.

Bethan and I used to fight over naming the various animals we had, which meant that we would frequently end up with some unconventional names. When naming our very first cockerel, we both took inspiration from our favourite films and TV shows. I loved any film about animals, of course. To this day my favourite film is *Lion King* and if you went to see the new live action version in the cinema recently, I was the adult man crying his eyes out when Mufasa died. My film of choice at the time was *Chicken Run*, in which the 'rooster' (bloody Americans) was called Rocky. My sister, on the other hand, was a big fan of *Only Fools and Horses*, thanks to our dad's influence, meaning that when our mum asked what she wanted to call the new cockerel, Del Boy was of course her choice. Rocky Del Boy was christened and then a few years down the line, Rocky Del Boy the Third arrived. Rocky Del Boy the Second, incidentally, after we'd asked a local farmer to source us a cockerel, turned out to be a Bantam. For those of you that don't know, Bantams are like the hobbits of the chicken world, and try as he might to have his way with our flock of full-sized, plump Rhode Island Red hens, come spring there were no little chicks. Safe to say he was quickly replaced by RDB the third. RDB the third, who was a superb White Sussex cockerel, about six months old, and, unlike his predecessor, absolutely gigantic.

Now I like to think I was born with an affinity for animals, but RDB the third really didn't want to be my friend. Every morning, bleary eyed, in the dark and cold, I would head out to the chicken enclosure with a pot of food and the hose to fill their water. I would get to the gate and no matter how quiet I was, he would be there waiting, his red eyes staring up at me. And as I approached, he would puff himself up and I swear he used to grow a full foot taller. I very quickly learnt that I needed some sort of defence when dealing with RDB the third and I found myself a large wooden board. I felt like a Roman soldier holding my shield out in front of me, parrying away his vicious attacks. As soon as my hand went on the door of the coop, he would start a low growl and then as the door opened his aggression would escalate to full-flung attacks – talons out, wings flapping, battering away at my pathetic wooden defence system. I must have spent hours being chased around the coop by that bloody cockerel, fearing that he would scar me for life with his sharp beak. I must admit I wasn't that upset when I came out one morning to find that the only bit left of RDB the third was his head, lying in the corner of the enclosure where the wire had been expertly lifted by a cunning fox.

My mum was the driving force behind my obsession with animals. She had always wanted to be a vet but never pursued her dream, and she quickly decided that it would be the perfect path for me. Everyone thinks their mother is the best but I'm afraid you are all wrong: mine wins. She was (and still is) hugely supportive and encouraging of everything I wanted to do, without ever pushing me to do anything. When I decided I wanted to work with animals, she helped me contact local farms, rescue centres and stables so that I could get hands-on experience with a huge range of animals. If I wanted to do something animal-related, she would do everything in her power to make it happen. She's a proper superhero.

I count myself incredibly lucky to have grown up in the countryside since it afforded me so many opportunities, which I would not have had in a city. From the age of ten I worked on a local farm, helping at lambing time and more often than not making dens in the straw bales. I had a school friend, weirdly also named Rory, who was a farmer's son. One of my happiest childhood memories is the two of us setting up those green plastic army men you used to be able to get, along one of the wooden beams of the big straw barn, and then shooting them down with bb guns or air rifles. I could also drive farm machinery from a very young age and learnt to reverse a trailer at thirteen, taught by my dad. I tell you what, it's not as easy as it looks!

When I turned fifteen I started volunteering at an amazing wildlife rescue centre called Oak and Furrows. It was run by the most incredible woman, Serena. She had started the centre in memory of her late daughter, and her passion for the place was fierce and unwavering. The centre was hidden in woodland near the lakes of South Cerney, a little haven of wildlife tucked away from the busy A419, and a mere half an hour's cycle ride away from my house. I loved the place as soon as I set foot on the site. I could be found helping with injured hedgehogs, pigeons, foxes, badgers and all sorts of other British wildlife to which I quickly became hugely devoted.

Lambing was always a fun time of the year, and I can't have been much more than eleven or twelve years old, sitting on the sofa watching some television before bed, when the landline rang. My mother answered and, with a tone of surprise, shouted to me to come to the phone. The mystery caller turned out to be the local farmer – he had a lambing ewe and needed my help. I was so flattered that I jumped straight on my bike and raced up to the farm. I had been helping him out for the previous few months, getting the barn set up for lambing and then helping feed and look after the lambs, once they started arriving.

The scene that greeted me that evening was of the mother-to-be sheep lying on her side in the floodlit barn. I had seen this done a number of times before and I wasn't afraid to get stuck in. I do wonder how many eleven-year-olds would be happy jumping straight in to help with lambing on a farm, but I didn't think twice and quickly dropped to her side. I remember it as clear as day, one hoof was sticking out of the sheep's vulva with what looked like a little black nose next to it. The sheep had been struggling for about thirty minutes and the farmer had been trying to help.

The farmer was a nice, kind fella – he had always been very encouraging of my love of animals and welcomed my help whenever I was available, especially as he was getting on a bit. Whenever I picture a farmer I see a rugged, thick-set, 6ft-something chap with rough spades for hands. Mr Douglas, as I knew him, was almost exactly the opposite. He was slight in build but strong as an ox, with piercing dark eyes behind ornate, tortoiseshell varifocals. He was a gentleman farmer. I'm sure through the years he had delivered thousands of lambs in a matter of moments, but these days it was a bit tricky for him. Farming is a tough job at the best of times, let alone during lambing season.

Having spent a lot of time on farms already, I had watched vets and farmers help deliver lambs and calves. Now, for the first time, it was my turn. I grabbed for a bottle of lubricant – industrial-sized bottles are commonplace on farms – and slid my hand up the side of the exposed hoof. The lamb's head was wedged against its front leg, its tongue sticking out about a centimetre from its lips. As I surveyed the situation I began to worry that I was dealing with a dead lamb. But just as that thought crossed my mind, almost as if it could hear me, the lamb gave a little flick of its tongue. It was subtle and weak but it was an unmistakable sign of life. I sped up – the head and one leg were pointing forwards but its other leg had been left behind, wedging the lamb in the mother's birthing canal. I had seen Mr Douglas and his sons deliver enough of these by now to know that this wasn't right: lambs were meant to be born with their two legs angled forwards alongside their head. I told Mr Douglas what I could feel and he explained that my only option was to lubricate around the head and push the lamb back in, to try to reposition it back in the mother's uterus. I quickly did just that and had the lamb back in the uterus in a matter of seconds.

The farmer watched on. 'You made that look easy, lad,' he said, as a word of encouragement.

'I think the mum is tired – she isn't pushing much,' I replied. Usually when you're trying to move an unborn lamb, or any foetus for that matter, around inside its mother, you fight a constant battle against the mother's strong pushes and contractions, trying to get you and their young out as quickly as possible.

I was now lying on the floor, perpendicular to the mother, up to my elbow trying to reposition the lamb. I felt around and grabbed on to the second front leg, then gently pulled it into the mother's pelvis to align the lamb. I think the sheep could sense that I had done what was needed because as soon as I had the lamb aligned, she gave an almighty push which expelled both my right arm and her lamb out into the big wide world.

The lamb flopped on the floor and lay motionless. I just sat up and watched, not knowing what to do. Thankfully, Mr Douglas stepped in – he must have dealt with this sort of thing hundreds of times; in a flash, he scooped the lamb up in one hand, using his other hand to poke a finger into the back of its throat to clear away all the goo that comes with birth. Then he started gently swinging the lamb backwards and forwards. He did this for about ten seconds, then laid it down and rubbed its body vigorously with straw. This process was one that I would come to use hundreds of times over the next fifteen years, and one that is cemented in my brain from that very evening.

The farmer and I crouched there, holding our breath, watching the lamb for any signs of life. The farmer was so calm. I, on the other hand, sat there anxiously looking at the lamb, then to the farmer and then back to the lamb like I was watching an odd game of tennis. The lamb coughed into life and started to shake its head – it was alive! I released my breath – I think I had been holding it for about a minute and a half. Mr D gently placed the lamb by its mother's head and, despite her exhaustion, she lifted her head and started to lick at her new lamb. It was a magical sight and I lay back onto the straw and closed my eyes. I wanted to remember that moment forever – this was the first life I had ever helped deliver and it was the best feeling ever.

I sat back up and said goodbye to the farmer, jumped onto my bike and pedalled home. As I walked through the door, I called out to my mum, excited to tell her the tale of my evening and was just starting to ramble when she said, 'Right, hold that thought, strip, and you can take that sheep shit from behind your ear as well!' Country living, eh?!

*

As a schoolboy you're meant to make friends for life. Well, someone forgot to give me that memo. I'm not sure if it was because I felt I understood animals better than humans, but I found making friends a challenge. Don't get me wrong, I tried, but I always felt more at home hanging out with four-legged species rather than two. I often wondered whether I would have been better suited to one of those posh boarding schools with a farm on site. But then I would have had to be away from my family, which would have been out of the question.

As well as animals, I loved two other things: cooking and sport. Cooking came from my mother, sport from my father. My dad had been a semi-professional footballer and school county champion at hurdling back in the day. He would have loved to work in sport yet ended up as a London businessman. I'm sure he enjoyed his job but he always preached to me to do something I loved. He got me playing football from a very early age and I ended up playing for a few teams through my schoolboy days. Sadly, I hadn't inherited my dad's natural talent, but God loves a trier. My dad and I would sit down every Sunday and watch Formula 1 and as many football games as we could, and when I decided I had had enough of football and preferred rugby, he started taking me to games at Bath and Gloucester.

I found school tricky (at least the social side) but I made do, working with a clear vision of where I wanted to be ten years down the line. I was never happier than at the wildlife centre, riding stables or on the farm, and that is where I spent most of my free time. When at school I used any opportunity to learn more about veterinary and the animal world, focusing my work experience placements and school reports around my future profession.

*

Being from the Cotswolds, when I finally got to start visiting veterinary surgeries to gain experience, I chose to spend a lot of my time in surgeries dotted around the countryside. The James Herriot-style of veterinary, seeing from puppies to shire horses and everything in-between – this is what I grew up fantasising about. But unfortunately the romanticised tales of veterinary practice in beautiful British countryside like the rolling Yorkshire Dales, with incredible stories of the most unusual characters, are a bit of a dying dream. The closest I ever got to this was driving around the Cotswolds, jumping from farm to farm, and I loved every minute of it. The Herriot books had always been a huge inspiration for me as a young boy and I have never felt, and probably never will feel, more connected to him than I did in those days. My parents had made sure to introduce me to the novels of Alf Wight (James Herriot was his pen name) as soon as I started to read. I think I must have read them all from cover to cover at least a dozen times, each time driving me further onto the veterinary path. He was soon my biggest idol, and a huge force behind my love for animals and veterinary. When I was twelve or thirteen, I went up to Thirsk, near York, to visit the Herriot museum and got lost amongst the historic equipment, photographs and incredible stories from the twentieth century. If you haven't seen it before, I cannot recommend strongly enough that you watch an episode of *All Creatures Great and Small*, the television adaptation of Herriot's stories. It is simply wonderful.

Over the years, as I said, this style of veterinary practice has passed me by, and city veterinary is what I have settled upon. It isn't what I had always dreamed of, but I have found my passion for it has developed and grown alongside me and my skills as a vet. I spend the majority of my time seeing cats and small breed dogs and I absolutely miss animals bigger than a spaniel, but, for now, I love what I do. As much as I love to think back to mixed animal practice with fondness, I can't help but be brought back to reality with a bump.

Times are changing massively in the veterinary world. It is the era of corporate veterinary, and vets are increasingly made to choose between pets, farm and equine work. As advancement after advancement is made in the medical field, both human and veterinary, the limitations of what we can do for animals are being reduced. We can do things in veterinary medicine nowadays that Alf Wight and his colleagues could only have dreamed of. With this, not only comes more knowledge and skills for the modern day vet to learn, but also a heightened expectation from clients that the vet should know everything about everything to do with their animal. With that overload of knowledge it is simply not possible to provide the high level of service expected from farmers, horse owners and pet owners if you are spreading yourself across all disciplines. As time goes on, the gap between the care we give our pets and the care we provide to humans is closing. I love nothing more than comparing notes with doctors on what treatments and latest technology they're using in human medicine and surgery. Inevitably, they always leave that conversation impressed with the level of care we give our patients. While at university, I had to make the decision as to whether to treat pets or farm animals. I love horses, don't get me wrong, but I could never see myself treating them. I ultimately came back to the animals I loved the most. It all started for me with my pets dogs and cats, so they are what I decided to dedicate my veterinary career and life to.

2

A Young Dr Doolittle

I wanted to be a vet from the age of four. My mum had been pestering my dad for years to get a dog. He wasn't the biggest animal man back then (you should see him now though!). He had never had a dog and he was definitely not like me with my love for all things great and small. I must admit I don't remember the exact way it happened, but eventually he gave in and one of my strongest memories from childhood is sitting in the car on the way to pick up our new puppy.

My mum had always wanted a Great Dane. It had all begun long before she ended up with my father, with a Great Dane called Heidi. She was the first Great Dane my mum ever met and belonged to a guy she had been dating. They lived in Cockfosters and my mum would go and meet her boyfriend in the pub. They would sit and have a few drinks, with Heidi curled up under the table. My mum would often head home before the rest of the guys (she always has been a bit of a lightweight).

The walk home was through a park, frequented by slightly dodgier members of society after dark. So Heidi would take my mother's hand gently in her mouth and walk her through the park like her personal bodyguard. Once home safe, Heidi would turn around and head back to the pub to join the rest of the gang. My mum, understandably, had felt completely safe and fallen head over heels with Heidi (less so her owner). Her obsession with Great Danes began and, twenty-something years later, that's exactly what we were getting. Looking back now, it was quite a commitment! If someone came to me with no experience with dogs and said they were going to get a Great Dane, I would probably tell them they were mad.

We were on the way to the breeder's house, we had picked the puppy out weeks ago and it was finally the day to go and collect her. I couldn't contain my excitement and we spent almost the entire journey discussing where she was going to sleep, how we were going to settle her in and, most importantly of all, her name.

As you'll remember from the incredibly named cockerel, Rocky Del Boy the Third, we each got a vote. My sister was only two or three at the time and she put up a huge fight for 'Miss Muffet'. These days, I see upwards of twenty pets a day in my job, and I have come across some pretty amazing names, but the thought of my mother or, even better, my father in the field next to our house shouting, 'Jesus Christ, Miss Muffet, just bloody come back!' starts me in fits of laughter. I like to think I got my choice because my suggestion was so far superior, but I'm sure it was simply due to the fact that my parents didn't want to name the dog after a character from a nursery rhyme. I had sat thinking in the back of the car for most of the journey and finally suggested

'Lulu'. To this day I have no idea where it came from – I must have been a huge fan of 1960s pop when I was four. 'Lulu' it was, and it was absolutely perfect.

We picked up Lulu at the tender age of eight weeks and had her until she was ten years old. That's quite a long life for a Dane and something I've always been quite proud of. When we picked her up she was all limbs, feet bigger than my four-year-old hands, with ears that drooped almost to the floor. She was everything I had ever dreamed of and I fell in love with her at first sight. She was a deep, rich blue-grey colour, known as a blue officially, something that I found hilarious as a kid. My friends used to ask what colour my dog was and I took great pride in announcing that she was blue, usually to my peers' disbelief – after all, who had ever seen a blue dog?

Once we got her back home to the Cotswolds, like any new puppy owners, one of the most important things my parents had to do was take her to the vet to get her checked over and start her vaccinations. I wanted to be involved in every small part of dog ownership, of course, so I announced that I had to be there for the first visit. I had never been to the vet's before but my mum already knew I had a love for animals that was special. There was a veterinary surgery at the end of the street where my grandmother lived. Every time we went to visit her I would ogle the masses of animals heading in and out of the clinic.

That weekend, we arrived at the veterinary surgery car park and got out with our little blue bundle of joy. My mum carried her from the car to the surgery – I was definitely not strong enough to carry her. Yes, she was a puppy, but at eight weeks she was already pushing the scales at a meaty 10kg, far too much for me. We found our way into the waiting room and took a seat among the bustling menagerie of dogs and cats. I could hardly contain myself with so many animals to say hello to, but I stayed put and dutifully cuddled our little pup – she was by far the cutest in the waiting room. 'Lulu Cowlam' came the shout from the vet's room – he had a northern twang which softened his bellowing voice. This is something that never fails to amuse people, whenever I'm chatting about my job with friends: they always chuckle that I have to come and call the pet's name in the waiting room. There are some incredible pet names out there: Captain Thunderpants (the puppy who used to wake himself up when he passed wind), Mr Meowgi (the cat that used to get a new fighting wound every week), Tinkerbell (the Rottweiler – one of my favourites), and, of course, Dave the cat (because who doesn't love a cat called Dave?).

We entered the room with Lulu and I got my first glimpse of a veterinary consulting room. It was a large, whitewashed room with high ceilings and laminate floors – very clinical, as you might expect. There was a single picture on the wall with a clock hanging above it. The picture was of a countryside scene and hasn't moved from that wall to this day. The centrepiece of the room was a large metal-block table with black rubber matting on the top – it was about as tall as me at the time. My mum walked in and popped Lulu down on the table as I stood in the corner and looked up at the vet. He had a huge presence in that room and I remember thinking I hadn't ever met anyone so in charge of everything. He held a hand out to my mother – 'Rod Benson,' he introduced himself. He had thick, dark hair, bright eyes and the tan of someone not shy to the outdoors. He had to be in his thirties at the time and was in great shape, the beauty of a physical job. He wore a checked, short-sleeve shirt and beige corduroy trousers with a white medical coat over the top.

We were in that consulting room for almost an hour, the first of many visits to come, and the conversation did not let up. Please don't be fooled, we spent about fifteen minutes discussing Lulu, and the rest was filled with topics such as growing up in Yorkshire as a child which, as it turned out, my mother and Mr Benson had in common, *Butch Cassidy and the Sundance Kid,* which was and still is one of Mr Benson's favourite films, marathon running, one of Mr Benson's casual pastimes, and finally the intricacies of classic cars, another passion of his. It was an awesome experience, though, and I sat listening in awe for the whole consult. Mr Benson got me involved – he let me listen to Lulu's heart through a stethoscope and he even showed me how to use the weighing scales to see how much Lulu weighed and then how much I weighed. It was amazing!

We said our goodbyes and left the vet's, Lulu having slept through her first puppy vaccination. My mum paid at the front desk and we ambled out onto the street towards the car. Now this is the part of the story I don't remember but my mother swears by it. As we left the vet's and the door swung shut, I looked up at my darling mother with my big blue eyes (yes, I told you it was my mother's story), and said, 'Mummy, when I grow up I want to be a vet just like Mr Benson.' And the rest, as they say, is history.

*

After that initial meeting, I saw Mr Benson pretty regularly. At the time we had the two cats, Creamy and Topsy, as well as Lulu, so we were regulars at the vet's and I was not one to pass up a visit to see my future mentor. I was the kid that made my mother make appointments after picking me up from school so I could go along – I loved the vet's! Soon we were familiar enough with Mr Benson to have a conversation about me spending some time in clinic with him and his team to see what the world of vetting was like from the other side of the consulting table. We had regularly discussed the fact that I had decided I wanted to be a vet, and Mr Benson was always encouraging and enthusiastic about my future career. When we broached the subject of work experience, Mr Benson made a point of telling my mother that he had recently stopped taking school students as they 'never got involved enough' and 'just stood in a corner and didn't make themselves useful', but both my mother and I assured him that I would throw myself in head first and ask all the right questions. He agreed, and I booked in a week to spend with him in the school holidays.

I was just turning fourteen and, by that point, I had known I wanted to be a vet for almost ten years. It's a weird one: veterinary – it gets under your skin; for me there was never anything else and it was such an early goal I had always just assumed that's how it was for everyone. I still remember when I was a young lad that friends, parents, teachers and any manner of interested adults would always ask the standard question: 'So what do you want to be when you grow up?' 'I'm going to be a vet,' was always my answer, and it was met with a mixture of reactions, but always with a look to my parents almost as if to say 'Well, he's damn sure of himself, huh?'

*

I must have been a few years into veterinary school when I was home for one of our infrequent university breaks. I was wandering around Cirencester, a town I had called home for a large portion of my life, and near where my parents still live. I was with my oldest friend James from primary school and we were just getting a coffee and having a catch-up. We had always been close; I couldn't tell you how many hours we whiled away playing football in the park or collecting the latest craze like Pokemon cards or Warhammer. James was now at Cardiff University reading Business and Economics – he was a bit of a business whizz and the course suited him. We were walking up from Starbucks and I caught a glimpse of someone I thought I recognised heading into Jessops. I told James to hurry up and we ran up to the window and gawked through. I was right: it was Mrs P – she had been our Year 4 primary school teacher, but had also taught us English.

I had always been a slightly hyper child and never stayed seated in class, but Mrs P found the right balance between respect and sheer fear, so I was generally a bit better behaved in her class. She had always taken a bit of extra time with me, and I had never really known why until she suggested to my parents that I was struggling slightly with English. She had her suspicions and wondered whether I could be dyslexic. At that time, there wasn't much help for dyslexic children but she was the first teacher to take enough interest to notice, and years later at university I was indeed diagnosed with dyslexia. She always had a big curly perm and a kind face with a sharp nose; she regularly wore a dress with a blazer, and that's exactly how she was on that day in Jessops. Our primary school had since closed down so I never had the option of going back to visit the place. I hadn't seen Mrs P since leaving primary school and I just had to say hello.

We waited until she had finished at the counter and, as she turned round, I said, 'I'm really sorry to interrupt but you're Mrs P, aren't you?'

'Well, well, well, Rory Cowlam, how are you?!' she said with some disbelief, looking me up and down. The last time she had seen me I had probably been about 4ft 10in, twelve years old with a pudding bowl haircut, and now I was nineteen or twenty and 6ft – quite a contrast (although still rocking an equally questionable haircut).

'I'm great, thanks, how are you? What are you doing with yourself now?' I asked, knowing that she couldn't still be at Ingleside.

'Well, I'm still teaching at a little place outside Ciren,' she replied (that's what the locals called it). We carried on the small talk for a few minutes – it was so nice to see her. 'Well, I must dash, the husband is waiting for me in the market-place. Oh, and Rory – ' she said, as she made to go, 'did you become a vet?'

'Yes, second year in training at the RVC,' I beamed back at her.

She looked at me and smiled, 'I knew you would do it.' And she turned and went on her way.

*

It's in Cirencester where you can find Mr Benson's veterinary surgery, and it was the summer holidays of 2006 when I was getting ready for my first-ever veterinary placement. I was fourteen at this point and I had spent years before then working on the farm, getting stuck in with cows, sheep, horses and pigs, but I had never worked as an actual vet. My mother drove me into Cirencester for 8am, and we pulled up in the car park of the old converted house. The building was two storeys: the ground floor was the vet's, with a few flats above. The whole thing was built of Cotswold stone – pale bricks stacked precariously, higgledy piggledy, on top of each other – unmistakable if you're from the West

Country. I jumped out of the car and said goodbye to my mum and went around to the front of the building. There was a plaque on the wall on the side of the entrance, one I had seen many times before, with Mr Benson's and his junior partner, Mr Babb's names and post-nominals written in bronze. 'I'll have those one day,' I thought as I pushed through the front entrance and walked into the surgery.

I was to spend a week shadowing Mr Benson and I was keen to get as stuck in as possible. I was soon getting a real taste of veterinary life, with consults in the morning, procedures, including X-rays, surgeries and dentistry in the middle of the day, and consults to finish off with in the evening. We even got out onto the farm on some days – it really was the mixed vet dream I had read about over and over again in the James Herriot books. My school had asked me to write about my experiences when I got back to class. I sat down to recount the highlights and decided to tell everyone about my Wednesday on the farm.

We had started the day by packing the car full of the essentials: wellies, waterproofs, buckets and brushes to clean ourselves, calving jack (a long device more reminiscent of something you would see in a torture exhibition at a museum rather than an implement to help deliver a calf), veterinary kit (including stethoscope, needles, syringes, thermometer, blood tubes and lots more), plastic gloves that came up to your shoulder, and drugs – many, many different drugs. We had set off in Mr B's old Jaguar E-type, not the most conventional of veterinary automobiles, but it did the job, and we pulled up at a large dairy farm in the middle of nowhere. It must have been over a mile down to the farm, across a bumpy, potholed dirt track. We parked outside a large barn which could have done with a little TLC: parts of the roof were falling off and the door was swinging off one of its hinges, a baby gate in its place. We met the farmer, Tom, a proper Cotswolds farmer. He was in a plaid shirt with dark blue overalls tied around his waist – he must have been mid-thirties, and had inherited the dairy farm from his late father. He was a big guy, but most farmers were to someone my age. He had a rough, grubby face with hands the size of my head, one of which almost took my arm out of its socket as he shook my hand.

'Not much to him, Rod – looks good for sheep, not these girls,' he laughed to Mr Benson, gesturing to the cows. Mr Benson, or Rod as he now was, looked round as he was grabbing his gear from the car.

'Don't worry Tom, you were his size once – we will make a vet out of him yet,' he replied. I smiled, hearing my mentor sounding so sure that I would be a future vet and hurried to get my wellies and overalls on. I must have looked a state, swamped by the vet practice's spare set of overalls, which I'm sure used to belong to Harry Potter's Hagrid.

We trudged through the makeshift baby gate door and into the dairy, my overalls down to my knees and dragging along behind me in the mud. There were ten cows lined up in crushes ready for us to examine. Despite the rather barbaric name, a crush is basically a large metal archway that the cow walks through, and then, when their head is in place, it closes just behind their ears to prevent them from moving backwards or forwards, as the farmer or vet is examining them. It most definitely does not crush them and, if anything, keeps both cow and human safe.

We were on the farm for what is called a 'routine' in the industry – veterinary slang for a regular, recurring visit to a farm. The vet sees any routine cases from the herd that wouldn't warrant an emergency call-out. Essentially, it's the 'general health check' of the farming world. On these visits, the vet usually sees issues such as pregnancy diagnosis, infertile cows and chronic illness. More acute injuries would be seen on an emergency basis, usually with the farmer calling up and asking for a visit that day or the next. I had never been on a farm visit with a vet before – I had only ever helped as a farmhand, getting the cows together for the farmer to put into a yard or crush for the vet to see. Mr Benson told me to grab a glove and asked Tom which cow was first.

'One on the end, thirty days, not sure she's in,' Tom said.

'Go on then,' Mr Benson motioned to me. I looked at him blankly – I had no idea what he wanted me to do, let alone what being 'in' meant. I tried to convey that in my facial expression rather than admitting it to the clearly sceptical farmer. Mr Benson picked up a bottle of lubricant, covered his gloved arm and threw it to me. 'Chuck some of that on and then copy me,' he said, taking a step towards the rear end of the cow. He lifted the cow's tail and then gently slid his hand into her rectum. He continued to insert his arm until his elbow disappeared.

'What you're feeling for is the pelvic brim. Once you're there, feel around and you should be able to grasp the uterus. If you feel something doughy like a leather football, you've gone too far.' Now there were a few problems with this: firstly, I had never performed a rectal examination on anything and, despite wanting to be a vet, it was still really gross. Secondly, I had no idea what a pelvic brim was and thirdly, no idea what a leather football felt like. Despite wanting to remind Mr Benson that I was born in 1992 and leather footballs hadn't been used since the 1980s I just smiled, mumbled 'Okay, great,' and lubed up my arm. To be honest I had learnt to expect this from Mr B; he always assumed I knew more than I did. Even to this day, as a qualified vet, I still feel incredibly inferior to him when we meet up and discuss veterinary life.

I walked up to the back end of the cow, lifted the tail and pursed my finger at its anal sphincter, which, as I made contact, tensed up as if to say, 'Not today, pal.' I began to insert my hand into the cow and in protest she started to whip her tail. Not preempting this, the tail slipped from my loose grip and smashed me straight across the face, leaving a trail of faeces like a pooey brand. I didn't look over my shoulder but was sure I heard Tom snigger. I grabbed the tail again and stepped towards the cow's rear end. This time I took a stronger hold and I gently pushed my hand in, the cow's muscular rectum closing around my wrist. It felt like submerging my hand in a warm sink of water whilst wearing a thin plastic glove. It was definitely a bit gross but I carried on, advancing my hand along the cow's colon, battling against regular, strong efforts by the cow to expel my hand and forearm from her bottom. I was shocked at how strong she was and kept having to re-find my footing to be able to push back against her. I felt the pelvis under my hand and moved slowly forward until I came to what I assumed was the pelvic brim. It was almost like a shelf which, once you felt beyond, led into the abdomen of the cow. At this point, I was almost shoulder-deep, my face worryingly close to the faeces-covered back end of the cow. I turned and looked at Mr Benson.

'I can feel the pelvic brim, and I think I'm in the abdomen,' I said proudly.

'Okay, so have a little feel around with a bit of a sweeping motion and you should be able to find the uterus,' he said in reply. There was no way I was finding anything in that cow: it wasn't pregnant (or 'in', as I finally realised what the farmer had meant), which meant I was fishing for a tiny uterus in a very large abdomen. I felt for another minute so as not to look disinterested or like I had given up, but really I was just grabbing at handfuls of liquid faeces.

'Okay, let me have a feel and we will see if she's in, Rory,' said Mr Benson. 'Bring your hand out slowly,' he continued, getting his arm re-lubricated. I carefully pulled my arm away from the cow. As I was about wrist-deep, she gave a huge push and expelled my hand at quite a speed. Not only did my hand return to the plain light of day but it was accompanied by a steady stream of steaming, liquid poo. Having not 'rectalled' a cow before, I was unaware that this was something that regularly happens when you are removing your arm. What you are meant to do is remove it in one swift motion to one side, ideally the side that neither you nor the farmer is standing. Unfortunately, I had pulled my arm away whilst standing directly in the firing line. The explosive faeces coated my front, splattering off me and hitting Mr Benson and Tom. Ordinarily this would have been a bit of a clean-up job, something you're faced with regularly on a farm and nothing a bucket of soapy water and a brush couldn't handle, but on this occasion I was in overalls seventeen sizes too big, so not only did the poo cover my front but, as if the cow was aiming, it fired inside the hanging front of the top and all over my shirt beneath.

I turned away, trying not to move so as to prevent liquid faeces from seeping into my boxer shorts and I whipped off my waterproof top and inspected the damage. My lovely pale blue shirt was now a mottled brown: essentially, I was a human cowpat. Mr Benson gave me a look of consternation, Tom was trying to stifle his laughter and I wanted the ground to open up and swallow me. 'Head back to the car, Rory, and give your shirt a clean in the bucket. Come back and find us when you're done,' Mr B said. I didn't need to be told twice and scuttled back to the car.

Later, I sat on a black bin bag as we drove back to the clinic, the Jag's windows rolled down the whole way. We didn't return to Tom's farm that week.

*

It was a bit embarrassing, but this was a story that my friends and classmates very much enjoyed hearing on my return to school. However, there was one other slight hiccup that week that really gave me a wobble about becoming a vet, one that I didn't really want to tell anyone about. We were in surgery on day one. We had spent the morning consulting and I had started to settle into the swing of practice life. My main take-homes from the morning's consults were: number one, vets seem to drink an inhuman amount of tea and coffee and number two, veterinary nurses run the show – they're the ones to butter up. I had just finished my fifth cup of tea and we were ready for the morning's surgeries. The day's list included a dental and two cat spays. Spaying is the colloquial term for ovario-hysterectomy – the removal of the ovaries and uterus from an animal – in this case, two lovely long-haired Maine-coon cats. I had kept making excuses all morning to spend five or ten minutes in the cat ward with the two sisters – they were adorable and loved a bit of fuss. I watched as the nurses prepared the first cat: they put her under anaesthetic through an intravenous catheter, placed a tube in her throat to allow her to breathe oxygen and the anaesthetic gasses and flipped her onto her back. They were clipping the belly of the cat from her ribcage all the way back to between her back legs as Mr Benson came in.

He explained to me that there were generally two ways you could spay a cat: through the midline, essentially along its belly, or via what's called a flank spay, an incision in the flank, or side of the cat. I tried to help in any way I could as I listened to Mr B; the nurses were like a well-oiled machine and the whole process moved very quickly. I had felt a little caught up in the whirlwind of the prep room – after all, this was the first time I had ever seen anything like this. We moved into the theatre, a box room with a big metal sink in one corner. Mr Benson was already waiting there in a sterile scrub top with his hands clasped in front of him, alerting the rest of the team that he was sterile and not to be touched.

The cat was placed in front of him and hooked up to an anaesthetic breathing machine. I was fascinated by the kit – it all seemed so high tech: there were monitors beeping, fluids running into the cat's vein and a bag that inflated and deflated with the cat's every breath. It was so cool and I wanted to know what every little thing did. I was told not to touch anything and stood dutifully, observing my mentor's every move. He covered the cat with a drape in one swift flick of the wrist – it fell perfectly, the hole sitting just over the clipped area that the nurse had prepared and, before I knew it, I was looking down at the insides of the cat. There was only a small amount of blood: blood had never phased me but it seemed odd, looking at the scene in front of me.

You couldn't really tell it was the same cat I had been play-ing with that morning. The green drape covered pretty much all of the cat except the area that Mr B was working on. It was as if the life underneath the drape was completely disconnected from the procedure in front of us. Mr Benson was chatting away, asking me questions here and there, tell-ing me the names of things as he fished them out of the abdomen and returned them to their rightful place. 'This is intestine, you see where the blood supply changes, that's where it turns from jejunum to ileum, now this big purple organ up here is the spleen, and then right over here we have the liver.'

He was just starting to fish out the first uterine horn and start the actual operation when the smell hit me. It was faint at first but it built as I concentrated more on it. Mr Benson's voice faded slightly as I tried to focus in on what was happening; the odd smell was like almost nothing I had ever smelt. The closest thing I could liken it to was raw meat slightly on the turn, mixed with the sterility of the operating theatre we were stood in. The smell of blood, the thick, heavy iron scent that I had become accustomed to having spent time working in a pub kitchen and a butchers. But even then there was something different, the fact that the animal was alive almost making it smell sickly sweet.

It all happened very quickly from there on in – my hands went clammy and my face flushed. My head felt like it was about to explode, my knees went weak and I thought I was going to vomit. Mr Benson had spotted my swoon out of the corner of his eye and called one of the nurses to come and help me, and she guided me out of theatre, sat me down and got me a glass of water. I looked down at my hands as I sipped the water – they were shaking and clammy. It took me a good fifteen minutes to recover. As I went back into the surgery, Mr Benson was just finishing. 'Feeling better?' he asked as I snuck in, sheepishly.

'Yes, a lot, thanks. I don't know what happened there,' I said, trying to laugh it off, but inside I was dying with humiliation.

'Don't worry, it happens a lot – at least you didn't faint and hit your head like the last one.' He laughed and gave the nurse a smile.

There have been a number of occasions in my veterinary journey which have really challenged my dead certain plan, and that was my first. I went home that day feeling stupid and weak, convinced I could never be a surgeon. Clearly I was squeamish and not cut out for the job. That's the problem with being so absolutely fixed on something being your future. I was so one-track-minded that anything that even vaguely threatened to set me back was devastating. There was no plan B: this was the plan and the only plan and it had to work. Looking back at it now, I can laugh about it – much bigger things have happened and having been in theatre pretty much every day for the last five years, I can assure anyone reading this that if you think you're squeamish from one experience, try, try and then try again. Some of the best surgeons I know started out a bit squeamish. I never did find out if Mr Benson was joking about the one that fell and hit their head, though.

*

By the time it came to thinking about university I already had a clear picture in my head of where I wanted to go, not that I had much choice with only seven universities in the UK offering veterinary medicine.

I will always remember the day I was accepted into the Royal Veterinary College. Veterinary medicine had been my goal for as long as I could remember, and that dream was slowly becoming a reality. When I opened my acceptance letter, I think my mother screamed at the top of her lungs for a full two minutes and I jumped in the air so high I hit my head on the ceiling.

When I had started down the line of applying to vet school, I had gone for a meeting with my school head of year, Mr Hills. He knew that I had always wanted to be a vet – it's hardly like I had kept it a secret – so as I sat down and he asked me, 'So Rory, what courses do you think you're going to apply to?' I should have guessed that he had other ideas. Mr Hills had never really liked me. Saying that, he had never really taught me; he taught German, and languages most definitely weren't my strong suit. I wasn't the most disruptive kid at school but 'wrong place, wrong time' was pretty much the story of my secondary school career. I was a smart student but common sense seemed to elude me as a teenager. I was always the first to offer to go and get the football from the roof or take a joke that little bit too far.

'Veterinary medicine, of course,' I replied matter-of-factly. There was never any other answer.

'Okay, but have you thought of other options? Veterinary is a really difficult course to get on to and even harder once you're there. I'm not sure you should put all your eggs in one basket.'

I nodded along – I had heard it all before. 'Yes, I know, Mr Hills, but I am going to go to vet school. I don't want to do anything else.'

This went on for weeks, no, months, and as I submitted my UCAS form to apply to four veterinary schools and no other courses (Nottingham, Edinburgh, Bristol and the Royal Veterinary College), Mr Hills called me into his office for the millionth time to have one final crack. 'Rory, we have discussed this at length, and I really think you should reconsider applying for only veterinary. It's quite unlikely you are going to be accepted.' He had stopped even attempting to be tactful from around meeting two.

'I know, you've said. Can I go?' I had also dropped the tact.

'Fine, but don't come complaining to me on results day when you don't have a university place,' he said, as I turned and left his office. I was going to show him. I was going to get into vet school if it was the last thing I did and then, then I was going to rub his smarmy, know-it-all face in it.

*

I got two interview offers from veterinary schools: Bristol University and the Royal Veterinary College. In all honesty, neither had been my first choice. When applying I had been to open days at the four I was leaning towards, and Nottingham and Edinburgh had really stood out. They were both super-modern, which I liked, and their approach to teaching seemed a lot fresher than the more traditional colleges at Bristol and London. I had always struggled to get the most from traditional teaching like lectures and seminars, and the innovative teaching at these more modern universities seemed like a really good fit for me.

As it turned out, Edinburgh and Nottingham declined my applications within the first few weeks after I had submitted. This was a huge kick in the teeth and I was starting to wonder if Mr Hills was right, but as luck would have it, Bristol and London wanted to see me.

On the day before my Bristol interview I was at work, in a local pub where I was a waiter, when I started to feel a bit off. I was sent home early, my manager commenting that I looked remarkably unwell. I didn't sleep a wink that night. I remember it clear as day: I was in cold sweats and kept getting up to have a cuddle with the toilet, worrying I would vomit. My interview was at ten o'clock in the morning. This was one of the biggest days of my life, so despite my mum's concern I got in the shower and put on my shirt ready for the big day . . . who couldn't beat a bout of food poisoning, huh?

There were bags under my eyes the size of small planets and I looked like I was going to collapse at any point as I bundled into the car ready to drive to Bristol. My mum nattered at me the entire way down the M5. I fired back monosyllabic answers interspersed with knowing grunts.

We eventually pulled up at the campus. It was huge compared to what I was used to at school and really quite daunting. The journey had taken just over an hour but it had felt like an eternity, and I stumbled out of the car as soon as we pulled up. I leant against a fence post and looked out over the field adjacent to the car park: there were horses grazing, a grey and a skewbald (I've always loved that name – it is essentially a fancy horse person's way of saying 'brown and white'). I must have looked like shit, doubled over in pain, unable to stand up straight and my face devoid of any human colouring, but I made my way to the reception area and checked in for my interview.

The interview was held in an old building – it could have been a chapel. With large stained windows and thick wooden doors, it was the kind of place that ordinarily would have been colder inside than out, the saving grace being a solitary electric heater they had plugged in to churn out some warmth.

I was called to the interview room and I made my way, looking like a modern day Quasimodo, off to face my fate. I had already come to terms with the fact that I was unlikely to excel at this interview so I wasn't nervous in the slightest – all I was focused on was trying not to be sick on the large mahogany desk between me and my interviewers. I apologised for my state, explaining my hunched nature and the interview started.

The interviewers were a bespectacled woman who looked a bit owl-like and very serious and, in complete contrast, a rugged farmer-type gentleman with a big, friendly face and boyish smile. I don't remember the interview in great detail but what I do remember is talking about rugby a lot, probably too much for a serious medical-degree interview.

I left, happy in the knowledge that I had not made a complete fool of myself, my stomach contents had not emerged mid-interview and I had clearly struck a chord with the farmer gent, who had failed to hide his joy at spending time talking about Gloucester rugby club instead of the usual foot and mouth or bovine tuberculosis outbreaks.

We pulled over on the hard shoulder on the way home, I leapt out and projectile vomited everywhere. I still don't know whether that was due to being ill or if it was a sort of nervous release. When we got home I lay on the sofa, popped the TV on and before long I was drifting in and out of sleep.

When I finally awoke, it was early evening. I spun my legs round and started to get up off the sofa. This was immediately followed by a searing pain in my abdomen, my legs gave way, and I found myself on all fours on the sitting room floor. I tried again to get up and slowly pulled myself up onto the sofa. I grabbed my mobile phone and called my dad; he was only upstairs in the office, but I didn't really feel like bellowing at the top of my lungs. He came downstairs, took one look at me and called the doctor.

We were at the surgery within fifteen minutes and the out-of-hours doctor immediately knew. She looked up at my dad and said, 'Right, so he has appendicitis. He needs to get to hospital ASAP. I can call an ambulance or you can drive him.'

My dad, it would be fair to say, is the most squeamish man on the planet, so the idea of an ambulance and hospital was most definitely not what he had planned for his Thursday evening. The ambulance would have taken a while to get to us so it was an easy choice to drive me straight to hospital. Hospitals, as you may have gathered, are not on my father's list of favourite places. I will always remember when he had to have surgery on his knee. He had injured it playing football when he was younger, his 'career-ending injury', and the only thing that prevented him from going on to be the next Eric Cantona. Much less glamorously, he was carrying some carpet down the stairs a few years later, only to slip and completely tear his ACL (anterior cruciate ligament) for the second time and bust his meniscus in the process. Surgery was recommended by his doctor and, after much deliberation, he conceded that it had to happen.

I knew my dad was squeamish but, until the day of his surgery, I hadn't quite realised how badly. He walked into the hospital and promptly passed out as soon as the nurse produced the IV canula. This time, however, it was me who needed surgery, so he chucked me into the passenger seat and drove me to Swindon General Hospital. That evening passed in a bit of a blur but one clear memory I have – and

I'll never forget – is looking over from the passenger seat and seeing what speed he was going. I have never been that speed since in a car and I don't suppose I will. Ever.

I had my appendix out that night, emergency surgery that no doubt saved me from a ruptured appendix and a horrendous peritonitis. The surgeon came round the ward once I was awake and told me how much of a close call it was. 'Another few hours and it would have burst, matey. You were lucky to get here when you did.'

I thanked him for removing the angry little organ that had been causing me so much pain. As he was leaving, he said, 'The nurses said you were rather lovely when you were recovering from anaesthetic. I think you told every single one of them that you loved them.' He gave me a wink and strode off down the corridor. He had such a presence – maybe I would be like that one day.

I only stayed in hospital for that day. By five o'clock I could stand and eat so they were happy for me to be discharged. As I was getting into the car to go home, my phone rang – a number I didn't recognise. I answered and immediately recognised the thick Bristolian accent on the other end of the phone – it was my interviewer from the day before. He asked how I was and I told him the story and explained I was just leaving hospital. 'Blimey, you've had a day, haven't you? Well, I just wanted to call you personally to say that we really enjoyed meeting you yesterday, even though you were in pain. You did brilliantly and we are delighted to offer you a place at Bristol Veterinary School.'

I could hardly believe it. Approximately 24 hours ago I was convinced I had flunked the interview because of my appendix. I thanked him and hung up. My first offer to vet school and all while my appendix was trying to kill me.

*

A few weeks later I was interviewed at the Royal Veterinary College. I had travelled up to London (which for a country boy was exciting in itself) to look around the Camden campus, feeling slightly more comfortable than the morning of my Bristol interview. The place was astonishing – everything I could have dreamt of and more. The thing that impressed me most was the museum of pathology samples, like what you might expect to find in the back rooms at the Natural History Museum. A full horse skeleton guarded the entrance: even that seeming mightily impressive to a young boy dreaming of one day being able to name and identify the endless rows of samples that lay before me. The interview went without a hitch, thankfully a lot less eventfully than the previous one, and I went home torn as to which university I preferred. I got an offer in the post a few weeks later, and I had to make the decision that would dictate the next five years of my life.

3

The Long Hours of Learning

I accepted the offer from the Royal Veterinary College and I'm absolutely sure I made the right decision. The RVC, as it's known, has been voted the best veterinary school in the world since I qualified, beating some pretty amazing schools. Everyone always thinks veterinary training is seven or eight years. I'm not really sure where that comes from, but if I had a pound for every time someone said, 'Seven years, isn't it? Longer than a doctor!' I would probably have a few hundred pounds to my name. I used to correct people, but now I just nod and agree – it saves the person immediately thinking less of you or, even worse, thinking that you didn't go to vet school after all.

You spend the first few years at vet school learning anatomy and physiology, essentially the building blocks of animals and how they work. This lays a platform for your clinical teaching in years three, four and five. But, as much as they tell you this, you spend those first two years asking, 'Why the fuck do I need to know this?', swiftly followed by a trip to the pub. At least, that's what I did.

*

Poo, wee, vomit, diarrhoea, pus, blood. You name it, veterinary professionals deal with it. Despite some early setbacks, once I was well and truly on my veterinary journey, there wasn't anything the animals of the UK could throw at me that I couldn't handle. I was proud to be well on my way to becoming a fully fledged member of the squad. If I look back now at the things I have dealt with over the years, it's a stomach-turning list to say the least. I've removed countless items from dogs' gastro-intestinal tracts (stomach and intestines), expressed the stinkiest of anal glands, delivered mummified foetuses, burst cheesy abscesses and washed out the most putrid uterine infections in cows (if you know, *you know* – it smells like death). The funny thing is, I can deal with it when it's an animal. If it was human poo or human vomit, however, there would be a Rory-shaped hole in the door.

Nope, humans are gross.

*

During vet school you spend countless hours shadowing experienced vets to learn the ins and outs of the profession. On one particular day back in my third year of veterinary school, I was working in Swindon, shadowing a young vet called Olivia. She was pretty, blonde and had the most incredible Irish accent – the clients loved her. She had only been a vet for a few years, but clearly loved what she was doing and always had a smile on her face. I don't know about other vets, but when I was a student I always gravitated towards the younger vets, and yes, it helped if they were pretty and female. I always felt the younger vets were more engaging on the whole, and took their time to help and explain things. After all, it wasn't long that they had been out in the big bad world of being a real vet, and they must have remembered what it was like being a lowly student stood watching consults in the corner.

We had just stopped for a coffee after surgery. I had helped in my first-ever bitch spay (removing the ovaries and uterus from a female dog) which, for any student, is a kinda big deal. I had walked to the staff room with my chin up and proud of myself. God knows why – looking back at it, all I had done was the easy bit, putting a few ligatures on where I was told to by the supervising vet. But never mind, I was going to take that win – I was basically a master surgeon now, right?

Over the years, one of the things I have enjoyed most is the shifting perception of my own achievements. I still see that sense of pride over super-basic surgery today while I'm teaching students. Don't get me wrong, it is absolutely warranted and completely deserved, but it isn't half funny looking back and laughing at yourself!

University is a bit of a lion's den at times, especially when you start your EMS (extra-mural rotations, or 'seeing practice'). After every placement block, there will be a ridiculous round of 'who did the most surgery' or 'who saw the coolest case'. I always tried to avoid getting involved in these 'one-up' battles – it just made people who hadn't done as much on a placement feel like they were behind, inevitably making them want to rush in when they eventually did get a chance to do some real surgery. I was hugely lucky with my placements in that they were surgery-heavy clinics, and they trusted me enough to let me get hands-on experience pretty much every day. But luck is exactly what it was. You trawl lists of veterinary practices when you're a student, trying to pick the ones that have decent surgical procedures, a nice practice 'feel', a friendly vet and vet nurse team, and one that isn't too far away from either your university acco-modation or 'home home', which for me was the Cotswolds. When I now have students come and shadow me, I make sure to try to let them get as involved as possible, just like the vets that taught me did.

*

Whether it was my way of trying to get 'one-up' on the other students or not, whenever I was in a practice, I always tried to find ways to set myself apart from the others. I'm sure this earned me the tag of 'kiss-ass' in vet surgeries around the country, but that didn't stop me. It might sound silly but tea and coffee has always been my thing, and I'll tell you why. When I was a young child, far too young to be holding a kettle and pouring boiling water, my darling grandmother taught me to make a good cup of tea. In her eyes, if you couldn't make a decent cuppa, you weren't worth her time.

The ironic thing is, she used to drink her tea like no human I have ever met: Assam tea bag, brewed to death with a drop of UHT milk. You won't be surprised to hear she also pretty much lived on a diet of Brussel sprouts and lemon cake. She was a woman of simple tastes, and one of the many incredible things she taught me was that if you want to endear yourself to anyone in life, remember how they like their tea and remember it. So, when I started visiting vet practices as a student, I made it my duty to learn every nurse and every vet's tea or coffee order and make them to perfection, and I tell you what, it always went down well – thank Grandma!

So inevitably, as Olivia and I made our way to start consults, I produced a cup of green tea with lemon for her. She gave me a wry smile and thanked me, muttering under her breath that she could definitely have made her own cup.

I'm sure all vet students end up doing this, but I also made sure that between every consult and pre every consult block, I gave the consult table a wipe down and cleaned up anything left out on the sides. Some vets are particularly organised, needles and syringes going in the sharps bins after every use, paper towels straight in the recycling, dog and cat hair swept up between each consult. Others, like Olivia, were not so tidy. I would dive around after her, picking up bits and pieces flying around the room – uncapped needles stuck into the rubber table top, ready for someone to stab their hand on – wiping pus from the abscess she just drained splattered up the wall and tea spilt over the side. Maybe the tea was karma's way of telling me to stop making it and sucking up. It seems table-cleaning is a long-standing tradition for vets and students, and has definitely continued to the present day with my own students rushing to clean residual wee, fluff or God-knows-what from the consulting table as I call in my next client; some, it must be said, are better at it than others. Only once have I made sure to take back control of 'table-cleaning duty' when, on calling in my new patient and spinning round to pop the cat carrier on the consult table, there was a thumb-sized nugget of poo smack bang in the middle of the table.

I set Olivia's tea down on the side, and dutifully set about cleaning the table and sweeping the floor. The clinic could only have been a few years old and still had a very new feel about it. In my opinion there are far too many vet surgeries out there stuck in last century, in converted townhouses with higgledy-piggledy corridors and miniscule consulting rooms. I admit there is something nostalgic and very James Herriot about these, but I like how clean and clinical a purpose-built small animal clinic can be, all glass and white walls: it just feels right to me.

Olivia walked out to the waiting area and called her next client in: she was a lovely old lady, Mrs Hoskins, with her slightly ageing cat Tibs. Now when I say slightly ageing, I mean he looked skeletal – to the point that he was struggling to hold his weight with his back legs. To be fair to Tibs, he did have some fight in him and gave a token growl as Olivia coaxed him out of his carrier. I translated the growl as meaning one of two things, either 'Watch my back – I'm a bit arthritic,' or quite possibly 'Oh not you again – just bugger off will you?' Either way, Tibs was not overly happy to be at the vet's.

'Okay Mrs Hoskins, I've got Rory with me today. He is a student from the Royal Veterinary College,' Olivia said, slightly shouting to compensate for Mrs H's hearing aid. She gestured to me, and Mrs H gave me a look up and down that only a distinguished older lady can get away with. It's a look that on the one hand makes you feel like a five-year-old boy at church dressed up in your Sunday best being inspected by the grandparents and stark bollock naked on the other.

'Lovely,' Mrs H concluded, and Olivia chuckled under her breath – clearly she was well acquainted with Mrs H's ways.

'So, how can I help today?' asked Olivia, beginning her consult with an open question just as they teach you at university.

'Well, Tibs is great as always,' Mrs H started, 'but he has developed a rather undignified habit.'

'Right, go on,' said Olivia eagerly. I think we were both starting to think this could be quite a laugh.

'Well, it's all rather horrid really. He has started leaving a bit of a smell behind him. It reminds me of rotting kippers!' she exclaimed in disgust.

'Right, well, that just won't do will it?! And am I right in thinking this is coming from his rear end?' asked Olivia.

'Oh yes, it's coming from his bum-bum,' she replied. No word of a lie, I almost spat my last sip of tea everywhere when she said 'bum-bum'. I turned my back and swallowed the tea down and had a little chuckle to myself as I grabbed some tissue from the dispenser, knowing what was about to follow.

'Okay, Mrs Hoskins, I think I know what's causing the problem. If you don't mind, I'll use Tibs to show Rory how to express anal glands – is that okay?' said Olivia.

'What glands, my dear?' asked Mrs H, in slight shock.

'Anal, Mrs Hoskins,' said Olivia, straight-faced and with no apology.

'Dear me, a girl of your age shouldn't be using such language,' said Mrs H. Olivia looked at me and gave me a smile. She must have known that would rile Mrs H as much as it did, and she clearly found my facial expressions of mild bemusement amusing, as she hid her chuckle with her reply.

'It's an anatomical word, Mrs Hoskins – everyone has one, eh Rory?' I blushed. I was used to observing, not chiming in on consults, but Olivia was clearly having some fun and wanted me to back her up.

'Um, well, yes, I suppose all animals have an anus,' I stammered, embarrassed to be caught between the vet and one of the poshest clients I had ever met.

'Well, do what you must, Olivia,' dismissed Mrs H, as she took a seat on the consult room chair. I was sure I saw the corner of her tight lips curling into a wry smile.

Olivia reached for an examination glove and some lubricant and I handed her the paper towel I was holding. For those of you that are not familiar with this delight, anal glands are two little broad bean-shaped glands either side of a dog's (or cat's) anus. They contain a putrid liquid that when released into the open, is reminiscent of month-old fish guts and can clear a room in less than three seconds. The function of these glands is to this day not one hundred percent understood, with some people believing they aid in lubricating the anus when passing a bone-heavy diet, but the running theory is that they are involved in scent marking and identification between animals. Safe to say that the secretions from these glands are generally God-awful smelling and if, like Tibs, the glands don't express and become blocked, they can be a right pain in the bottom. The glands are located at about four and eight o'clock if the bum hole were a clock face, and one of every vet's favourite jobs is to pop a finger in an unassuming animal's anus and express the blocked glands like milking a grape. For those of you not versed in sarcasm, that was a prime example and I must admit as a qualified vet, it seems that all my anal gland appointments seem to get booked in first thing in the morning, or right after lunch – maybe my receptionists just really like the idea of me having to run to the prep room to vomit up my hastily finished sandwich. Expressing the glands themselves is a relatively swift and easy procedure in a well-behaved animal.

Don't get me wrong – it can't be terribly comfortable having a human's finger inserted into your rectum and gently squeeze a full gland in your anal sphincter, but generally most animals are very well behaved with this. Even so, I always get a second person to hold the animal as I do it because, if they wriggle, this seemingly easy procedure can become a bit of a palaver.

In this particular instance, Mrs H was having none of it and I don't think she would have held Tibs if Olivia had been so brazen as to ask. She was busying herself in the corner of the room, trying very hard to remain unassociated with whatever was going on with her darling Tibs's bum-bum. Equally, Olivia was trying her hardest to show me exactly how to express the glands, so we ended up with me holding Tibs on the table, cuddling him to my chest, while Olivia talked me through it. She lubricated her finger – 'No such thing as too much lube,' she said with a smirk, loud enough for Mrs H to hear. 'So you just slip a finger in and feel for the gland and once you have . . .' Tibs let out quite a groan mid-sentence, interrupting the vet mid-stride.

Now, all of you reading this have said the word 'have' at some point, or another in your lifetime. If by some miraculous turn of events, you haven't, please make the motions now. You will realise that as you enunciate the 'aaaa' sound, your mouth opens rather wide. Well, it was at this exact moment that dear Tibs decided that he had had enough of this human finger in his bottom, and he tensed his anus while letting out a heartfelt yowl, that I can only assume translated as 'fuck you'. The bit I missed, as I looked quizzically at the ageing cat, was that as this happened, the pressure in Tibs's anal gland reached critical point, producing a stream of foetid juice which flew through the air and landed perfectly on the back of Olivia's tongue. For what felt like a full minute she stayed put, kneeling at the side of the consult table, mouth open like she had suddenly developed lock-jaw. The look of horror on her face was a picture and, as what had happened fully dawned on her, she dived head first towards the consult room sink. She just about managed to get over it before her stomach caught up with her thought process and promptly emptied its entire contents, including a few wonderful sips of green tea with lemon, down the drain.

At this point Mrs H looked up in disgust from her perusal of the week's events in her diary which she carried in her Gucci handbag, 'What on earth is going on?' she exclaimed. I looked round at Olivia, head first in the sink, and tried to formulate an explanation in my head that would satisfy Mrs H, but quickly decided that it would be easier to tell a white lie and move on.

'It looks as if Olivia has been taken ill, I'm afraid. Why don't you go and have a cup of tea in the waiting room and I will come and find you once we have everything sorted.' I offered Mrs H an arm as I escorted her from the room and then returned hurriedly with a glass of water to Olivia. She didn't look in a good way and was frantically trying to scrape all residue from her tongue. I think she was probably weighing up the pros and cons of cutting it out of her mouth. She sat on the floor and continued to swill her mouth out. I picked up Tibs and sat down with her, stroking the cat who now seemed quite settled on my lap, clearly rather proud of himself.

'Well,' she finally said, 'that's never happened before.' I must admit, I'm not sure there are many things worse than anal glands, especially when making a list of things I really wouldn't like to know the taste of. The smell is bad enough – Mrs H really was right with her rotten kipper comparison. Sitting there, I detected a faint odour of week-old fish. I wasn't sure if it was Olivia or Tibs but decided it was probably best not to ask.

I have heard of many anal gland mishaps over the years. One of my friends once told me the horror of emptying an Irish Wolfhound's anal gland, the size of a small tangerine. He managed to spray the contents, sprinkler-style, all over the owner and their nine-year-old daughter. Still to this day though, I am yet to hear of another vet expressing a gland into their own mouth. I learnt a very important lesson that day and, as you are reading this, let this be the one thing you learn from me. Never, and I repeat never, have your mouth open while expressing an anal gland.

*

Once you spend enough time in a clinic, you really start to feel at home, and that's exactly what happened with me at Olivia's practice. I felt like one of the team. I was handed an iPad every morning on my way in (as I said, it was a very fancy modern clinic) and it had 'Rory's consult list' on it, which inevitably was another vet's list but I was to run it. So, I would start the consult, take a history from the owner, examine the pet and then go to present my findings and plan to John, the head vet of the practice. John would then swan in, double check that I wasn't being an idiot and then tell me to carry on. It was a great system – it meant that John could sit and do all his paperwork while I learnt, very quickly, how to run a consult. I saw everything from limping dogs to vomiting cats, and learned how to give vaccinations properly and, most importantly, how to talk to clients. It was terrific experience.

No-one ever tells you that veterinary won't be all about the animals. You spend your whole life wanting to be a vet, training for years and years in order to help the animals, and then you very quickly learn that it isn't just the animals – you also have to speak to the general public and, oh dear me, that can be tricky. When I was applying to vet school in 2009, I remember being sent questionnaires by the veterinary school admissions teams asking what I thought being a vet was all about, and what I imagined the good things and bad things about the job were. I always got my mother to read through my responses before I sent them off as I valued her opinion massively, and I suppose I also lacked tact at times. She called me one morning and I wandered into the kitchen to find her in fits of laughter, reading through my application. Where the question had asked, 'What is the worst thing about the veterinary profession?' I had written, 'The clients'. At seventeen years old, I had thought it 'tongue-in-cheek' with an undertone of truth. She made me change the answer, and yes, that may be one of the reasons I am sitting here writing this book today.

*

It was a normal mid-week day, I had started my morning consults in the standard fashion, putting on my most grown-up voice and trying to pretend I knew what I was doing. I learnt very quickly that there was a benefit to having a bit of stubble on my face; at the time I was only 21 and, if clean shaven, regularly got doubtful looks as I called owners into the consult room. These looks were inevitably followed by comments such as, 'Don't I get to see a real vet?' Consults then went without a hitch, except for the usual baby-face jokes from clients. Anyway, that day I was actually quite proud of myself for diagnosing Sarcoptes Scabiei in a spaniel by doing a skin scrape and, looking under the microscope, seeing horrible alien-looking things crawling all over the glass slide looking for some skin or blood to eat.

When I had finished, I wandered through to the prep area with a coffee – it was my favourite time of day: surgery time. We had a list of five procedures that day and I had already missed a few that morning, but there were two cat spays left to do. Removal of the uterus is a routine procedure in cats and dogs. This is one of the things I discuss at length with my clients nowadays. In particular, in dogs it is quite a big procedure and often owners are very tentative to put their dog through it – understandably. There is also an ongoing debate about when to actually carry out this procedure, whether before or after the dog comes into heat for the first time. It can be a really difficult decision for owners. In cats, however, it's a bit more of a no-brainer.

When cats come into season they start 'calling'. 'Calling' is exactly what it says on the tin: the cat becomes very flirtatious with everyone and everything in its path, including inanimate objects such as arms of the sofa and chair legs. Besides this amorous behaviour, they start wailing –wailing through the day and night, keeping all in the house awake and driving you up the wall. It is no wonder then that I regularly get calls from people with cats around eight months old requesting an emergency spay booking, often despite me warning them of this when seeing them with their new kitten six months previously. I must admit, I take great joy in making these people wait another few days before we can book the cat in – we want the cat to be slightly calmer before doing the spay anyway.

The operation can be done in the flank or the midline; the flank operation is the most widely used approach and the procedure itself consists of a small incision, around a centimetre long in the left side of the cat. The incision is made just in front of the back leg muscles, to act as a window into the cat's abdomen which allows for identification of the uterus and ovaries. The surgeon then places ligatures (encircling knots to occlude blood vessels) on the ovaries to then remove the whole reproductive tract as one. When you are training as a vet and shadowing experienced surgeons, this operation is one of the first four operations you endeavour to learn. The 'routine' operations include castrations and spays of both dogs and cats.

I was excited then that there were two young kittens in the ward waiting for their spays. I had tried to follow a kind of mantra with any practical skill: watch one, do one, teach one. It was a great way of making sure you understood fully how and what you were doing. I had seen a few cat spay operations before but never done more than a few little bits of the procedure, and when I had seen these two on the board that morning, one of the vets, Dan, had said I could watch him do the first one and then we could do the second together, start to finish. The cats were gorgeous, no more than about six months old, their coats a blend of rich caramel, silver and pure white. I was giving them a little bit of fuss when I heard Dan call in, 'We are good to go, Rory.'

I scooped up the nearest one – she was called Petal and had beautiful blue eyes that were slightly covered by her third eyelids (yes, cats and dogs have a third eyelid that moves across the eye rather than up and down). The pre-op medications had made her all sleepy. She cuddled in under my chin as I walked her through to the prep area and I put her down gently on the table. Dan let me place the intravenous catheter and induce the anaesthetic. I placed the endotracheal tube (breathing tube) into her throat and she breathed deeply, moving deeper and deeper into the sleepy realms of the anaesthetic with each breath. She was placed onto her side, and the nurses swept into action, clipping, prepping and sterilising the surgical area. Dan and I moved into the theatre and started scrubbing our arms and hands like you do with any operation. Dan was quite a sporty guy, loved his football, so we caught up on the weekend's results – Arsenal had absolutely hammered West Ham and Dan was a huge Arsenal fan. I asked him basic questions about the operation and then about him as a vet. I was always interested in hearing about people's paths to veterinary – no two stories were ever the same. He was a recent graduate, just over a year qualified and had spent six months working in a mixed animal job before moving to small animals only. He struck me as quite confident for a relatively newly graduated vet, but then everyone seems confident when you're a student.

We finished scrubbing and I grabbed a paper towel from the dispenser in front of me to dry my hands. 'What are you doing?' asked Dan as he saw me blotting the water from my arms. I turned to look at him and his face had gone all serious, like I had just been caught doing something unspeakable. I looked down and saw Dan with his sterile hand towel. 'Shit,' I thought. I had been on autopilot and dried my hands with a normal towel, essentially undoing the last five minutes of hand washing. 'Do it again. You can join me when you're sterile. Tori, keep an eye on him, please,' he said to the nurse in the room. She looked at me and gave me a wry smile. What an idiot I was. You spend your whole time on placements trying not to make stupid mistakes like that and I had just been a grade A plonker. I must add, I didn't use that opportunity to tell him I had done exactly the same thing a few mornings prior to castrating a cat (oops). It was fine, I saw the cat again a week later and it had healed beautifully – no post-op infections in sight. I re-scrubbed under Tori's watchful eye, trying to laugh it off, making sure I now used a sterilised hand towel.

I was putting my gloves on when I heard some commotion from theatre – something wasn't right. 'Tori, get John, NOW!' Dan's voice was fraught with panic. I peered through the theatre door window – what could have gone wrong? Dan stood there, his hat and mask obscuring most of his face, but I had seen panic before and I could read it in his eyes. He was frantically fumbling with instruments on his surgical tray with his right hand, his left outstretched holding a bundle of swabs onto the side of the cat. Despite the frantic nature of the surgeon, everything else seemed normal: the nurse sat monitoring the anaesthetic, there was no blood spurting up the wall or pooling on the floor, the cat was lying motionless and the breathing bag on the anaesthetic machine was still rising and falling with each breath. I slowly entered the room and was just starting to offer my help when John came bursting towards the door.

'What's happened?' he asked, quickly starting to scrub his hands and arms.

'I don't know,' Dan replied shakily. 'There is just a lot of blood!' John threw some sterile gloves on and dived straight in. He glanced in through the incision Dan had made, had a quick look and then started conducting his team like an orchestra.

'Okay, we have to go midline, I'll stitch this, get some clippers and a quick prep for the abdomen. Jo, watch her like a hawk and let me know if she starts to destabilise.' It was controlled chaos, he had the cat closed within a minute and then the nursing team flipped the cat onto her back, clipped up her fur and quickly prepared her skin to be sterile. Within just three minutes, John had come in and taken control of the situation. The tension in the room was thick and I tried to slink away into the corner. I knew it was important to see these things – you need to know how to react when things go wrong in surgery – but, as a student, the worst thing you can do is get in the way.

John started to open the cat's abdomen along the midline in one bold cut with the scalpel blade. He popped through the peritoneum, the final layer when going into the abdomen, and suddenly everyone in the room took a simultaneous gasp. Blood poured out from the cat's belly in a crimson waterfall, flowing over the drapes and down onto the floor, splattering everywhere as it sluiced onto the marble tiles. 'She's getting weak,' Jo, the nurse watching the anaesthetic piped up. Releasing that amount of blood from the abdomen meant the cat likely had very little left. I stood in the corner and watched; I could do nothing to help, and considered trying to leave them to it but my feet were stuck to the floor – I couldn't move. I was hardly involved: I hadn't even been in the room when it happened, but I was as tense as I had ever been in a veterinary situation – it didn't feel real. All I could really focus on was the beep, beep, beep of the pulse oximeter, tracking Petal's pulse and watching as more and more blood flowed from the little cat's abdomen. The beeping of the machines suddenly changed – 'Is it me, or is that getting slower?' I thought to myself, making the decision that it would have probably been quite unhelpful to point that out in the middle of the emergency situation. Indeed the beeps were getting more spaced out, and after about half a dozen slow blips, they faded into silence. 'She's gone,' said Jo.

'I just can't find the bleed,' said John. 'Start IPPV*, Dan, start compressions,' John was cool and collected despite the horrific situation in front of him, and I couldn't help but be hugely impressed. 'I want to be like that someday,' I thought.

Petal died that day. She had come into the clinic early that morning, just six months old, healthy as anything with her sister and, just five hours later, she was in a body bag. I had seen pets die before but never due to a mistake, never because something went so catastrophically wrong. I had seen vets get emotional before – it was so clear at times – but that day I saw the real toll the job could put on you. Seeing an otherwise healthy animal die was a really indescribable experience – in reality it was quite humbling. We as vets try to do what is right for animals but that was a true reminder of how delicate life is. It hangs in the balance and at any moment, with a simple mistake, the worst can happen.

* IPPV is 'Intermittent Positive Pressure Ventilation' – essentially breathing for the cat. It is something you occasionally have to do in surgery if an animal will not breathe for itself, but it is also a core part of CPR or cardiopulmonary resuscitation.

Dan was, as you can imagine, distraught. After the team conceded that Petal was gone, he walked out of the room and disappeared. I asked John if there was anything I could do and he told me to help tidy, so I did. After a crisis like that, staying busy and keeping the clinic functioning as normal can be hard. Often if you stop to think about what went wrong, it can put other patients at risk. Dan eventually emerged – he had obviously been crying: his eyes were bloodshot and his face was puffy. He looked ill: it was as if his eyes had sunk into their sockets – they had most definitely lost the sparkle they had had that morning. He asked if John was around and then went off to find him, sniffing, trying to make it seem as if he was okay. I picked up a bundle of towels and blankets and walked down the corridor towards the dog kennels to put them away. I stopped just outside the kennels – John and Dan were inside. I listened for a few minutes to what they were saying; Dan was understandably devastated. John had worked out that Dan's approach had been too far cranially (towards Petal's head end), and he had cut into the kidney and nicked an artery, a simple mistake with huge repercussions. The added complication here was that Petal's sister, also in for the same operation, was in a kennel waiting for her turn and Dan had to work out what he was going to do. I walked away, not wanting to be caught eavesdropping. I did not envy Dan.

I didn't hear the conversation between Dan and the owner but I can only imagine how hard that would have been. He came back after the call with the owner's consent to perform the next op on Petal's sister. I don't know to this day how he managed that one but, as you probably could have guessed, John made sure to be in the room as Dan started his approach. He didn't say anything, just watched. This, I thought, was good management: he was there when Dan needed him, but allowed Dan to carry on and learn from his mistake. I know it must have been hard for Dan, but I wonder how many vets would have done the same as John that day. It was his business, his reputation on the line here, and Dan could very easily have made the same mistake again on the second cat. It must have been really hard for John to let Dan crack on and not intervene. The second op went smoothly, without any issue. Dan's hands had been shaking at the start but once he found his rhythm, he was back to being the confident surgeon he was before, almost. John left halfway through, once he knew Dan would be okay and I stood and watched, slightly disappointed that I didn't get to do one of the spays, but thankful that it wasn't me who had been doing Petal's. That must have been one of the hardest things to go through as a young vet.

Now I'm a fully qualified vet, five years in, I look back at these things with dread. Being a recently graduated vet is one of the most stressful things. I recently spoke to Linda, John's business partner and Dan's other boss. I hadn't heard from her for a few years and she was actually enquiring to see if I wanted a job – oh, how things have changed! When I had spent time at her clinic seeing practice, she never really got involved in teaching or going through cases with me. Luckily, John was much better at it than she was – he was a born teacher. He had really invested a lot of time in me. Linda had hardly been around but when she was, she paid little attention to me. I got the impression over my time there that she probably thought I was a bit of a waste of space because I wasn't one of the 'smart' students. She was quite a harsh woman and I was more than a bit scared of her. So much so that whenever she asked me to do something, I inevitably made a mistake or didn't do it quite right. Linda wasn't one to give more than one chance and she had quickly written me off.

At one point while making me work out a drip rate for a medial inpatient, she had said, 'You're not the smartest in your year, are you?'

I had been a bit taken aback at the brazen nature of the question. 'Well, I suppose I'm not that book smart, Linda, no.' She had come to the conclusion that I had charmed my way into vet school and didn't really deserve to be there, so years on when we bumped into each other at a veterinary conference, I was surprised she remembered who I was, let alone offered me a job. I politely declined, saying I was happy with my current position but exchanged details with her as a courtesy. As we were parting, I doubled back and called after her, 'Linda, I just thought I would ask, what's Dan doing these days?'

'Oh,' she replied, 'Dan left a few months after the spay incident. I think he was struggling with the pressure. He isn't a vet any more – I think he is back home, farming.'

This and so many other stories like it are all too common. Dan had spent five years training to be a vet, and he had spent his first six months in a job working insane hours trying to find his feet as a new graduate. He had reached breaking point in that job and made the decision to move to a different kind of practice altogether, where he started to feel more comfortable and get into a rhythm. But a mistake here, an angry client there and building pressures eventually ended in him reaching the point of no return. He left the profession within two years of entering it, less than half the time he spent training to to be a vet. Now don't get me wrong, his degree is not wasted – he has some very valuable letters after his name and will no doubt use the knowledge and experience he has to great effect in whichever job he ultimately ends up in, but this was my first insight into the true pressures of being a vet.

To this day I still think of Dan. I still remind myself of how tough being a vet is and how privileged I am to be in a job where I am supported by amazing colleagues and excellent bosses. I am all too aware that this isn't the case for a lot of vets. Fortunately, though, times are changing. More support mechanisms are starting to be put in place for young vets and the profession is coming together to look after its own. It is a wonderful thing to see and I wonder if Dan had been in the profession now, whether he would still be working as a vet, or was he simply not meant to be one.

4

The 'Q' Word

I think all in all I observed practice at about ten different clinics over the course of my training. I made sure to get a wide variety of experience, from charity clinics to the Herriot-style mixed practices, to the most high-tech referral practice. There is a huge amount of variation in the veterinary world, more than you would think. If you consider everything one can do with a veterinary degree it can be mind-boggling. Just from my group of university friends, there are farm vets, small animal general practitioner (GP) vets, surgery interns, surgery residents, medical residents, cardiology residents, equine surgeons, an ophthalmologist, an emergency and critical care specialist, a neurologist, two chicken vets (yeah, even I don't know how I know two guys who became chicken vets), pharmaceutical reps and one who works at the Home Office. Safe to say, that's some pretty good variety all from one degree, and that's not all of it! There are countless opportunities in research, government work, and even abattoir work as well as the more conventional routes. I have spent the vast majority of my time with small animals, pets essentially, but I have seen or experienced most of these avenues and could have ended up going down any one of them. No, before you start, I have never been to the Home Office and, trust me, I would have made a terrible chicken vet. I chose small animal veterinary for one simple reason: my love of dogs.

From what I have seen across the world of veterinary, there is one quite hilarious common thread that runs through the industry. It was instilled into me from a very early point in my student career, quite possibly the first time I ever set foot in a practice as a vet student. You may not quite believe it but the veterinary industry is full of superstition, and no, I'm not joking. I have often wondered about superstition even though I myself am a complete sceptic and stories of ghosts, ghouls, freaky happenings and 'tempting fate' just aren't for me. The people in the veterinary industry are generally intelligent people of science, and surely as people of science we do not believe in such hokum?

Wrong! I can guarantee that both the human and animal medical professions are rife with superstition. Me included. Those of you who watched as many *Scrubs* episodes as I did over the last ten years may remember Turk and his lucky doo-rag . . . that's now me. I have fallen victim to having a lucky scrub cap. Now I know as well as the next person that my surgical outcome will not vary depending on which patterned scrub cap I have on my head – my Batman one, my Superman one, my Pacman one, my Star Wars one or my one that looks like a brain – but then again, will it? If I wear my lucky scrub cap, and, yes, it varies from time to time (as I write I'm having a rather good run with Batman), I feel more relaxed as a general rule. Surely then, the relaxation that comes from having my lucky scrub cap tied upon my head leads to a more relaxed and careful approach in my surgeries? Can you not then see a link between a more considered approach and my choice of headwear that day? Too far?

Okay, well how about this: there are a number of studies out there that show a happy and friendly surgical team (i.e. the surgeon, the assistant, the nurses, the anaesthetist and so on) that communicates well, has a statistically better surgical outcome than those who do not know each other and do not communicate effectively. This was so strongly proven in one case that an anaesthetist from Australia started to embroider his name and job title on his surgical scrub hat, meaning everyone knew who he was and why he was there. It was even suggested that this started to improve outcomes of emergencies such as cardiac arrests, as everyone knew who each other was and could communicate more effectively and clearly rather than just pointing and calling each other 'you' or 'hey' or 'doctor'. By no means am I suggesting that my comedy scrub caps will help with that sort of thing – after all we work in a much smaller team where everyone knows each other well – but if I am wearing a funny scrub cap that lightens the mood, especially in an intense and serious surgery, it isn't beyond the realms of possibility that it may help morale and therefore the outcome for our patients. Right, well, that's how I justify my obscene number of scrub caps to myself, and also how I explain my occasional sense of humour failure if I don't have the right cap for the job.

There are two superstitions that cling to the veterinary profession more than any. I am sure that any veterinary professional reading this will know what I'm talking about when I reference the 'Q' word. In fact, I'm sure this must translate to a huge number of industries. I can almost feel veterinary prep rooms around the country shuddering at the very thought of someone walking in and exclaiming for all to hear that it's looking *quiet*, or how *quiet* it has been this week, or suggesting that it's going to be a *quiet* day. I learnt this the hard way, walking into one of my first placements after lunch, and saying to the nursing team busying themselves discussing last night's *Love Island* gossip, 'Bit of a quiet one today, isn't it!' A roll of bandaging material, a capped (thank God) syringe and a 500ml fluid bag came flying at my head.

'Do not use the Q word,' hissed the head nurse, 'or YOU will be staying to deal with the consequences,' and, dear Lord, she was serious. I'm afraid I still don't buy into this one – after all, I'm someone who much prefers to be busy than quiet, but even I have been worn down over the years. You won't find me even entertaining the idea of saying the 'Q' word at work; it's just not worth the repercussion. I know people who have seriously fallen out over it!

Secondly, there is 'Friday Night Syndrome', a phenomenon that I'm sure some of you will be aware of. Now I suppose this isn't really a superstition – it's more of an idea or theory. The theory is that no matter how 'quiet' (sorry guys) your week has been, you can guarantee at least one emergency call as things are starting to wind down before the weekend. I'm sure the same goes for those of you working in offices, where you get a pile of work dumped on your desk at five o'clock on a Friday. I was discussing this with a receptionist I work with and she was trying to convince me that it was a real thing. 'Honestly, five to seven, on the dot, that phone will ring,' she exclaimed, pointing at the phone. I bet her a glass of wine that evening that it wouldn't and went about my day I love being sceptical about these things as I am most definitely in the minority, and everyone wants to prove you wrong.

At a quarter to seven I went back to reception to make a coffee. It had been one of those days, slowly ticking along, dragging that little bit too slowly right up until evening consults, and I was a bit taken aback as I clocked the time. 'Blimey, five minutes ago I was starting evening consults,' I muttered, and since then I had seen a bleeding dog, a cat with an eye ulcer, a recheck on my favourite Labrador from last week who had thought it was a great idea to eat a tennis ball whole and a terret that needed its nails clipping. I really do love how varied our profession is . . . Anyway, it was coming close to closing time and so far no emergency. I had that internal dilemma as to whether to start gloating to the receptionist now or after five to seven when I was definitely in the clear, but who was I kidding, I couldn't help it: 'Looks like I was right,' I mumbled as I wandered past. She just rolled her eyes – I could see her almost begging the phone to ring.

I returned to my consult room to write notes and finish my coffee. That is one thing that five years of university and a career in veterinary almost guarantees: you will learn to drink coffee at all times of day to keep yourself sharp. To put into perspective how important coffee is to me in my clinic, when I was in my first job, my boss came to my branch for our quarterly review. I had been there for three months running a quiet little branch practice as a bit of a break from night work. It was a little shop front, designed as a consulting-only clinic, with one receptionist and me as the vet. The idea was to feed business into the big hospital where I also spent a lot of my time working overnight. We were incredibly quiet compared to the busy hospital, but it was a nice change from the constant go, go, go. I couldn't tell you a single thing she said in that review, except for her surprise when I offered her a coffee from the Nespresso machine I had purchased for the clinic with my first pay check. She had given me a quizzical look and I had simply replied by saying, 'The dogs deserve me on form.'

So there I was, sitting in my consult room with my coffee, trying to remember the heart rate of the cat I had seen three hours ago, typing up my clinical notes from the day. I heard the phone ring and prayed for it not to be an emergency. I peered round my consult door and my receptionist looked at me, her eyes lit up. 'Damn,' I thought, she was right.

'Bring him straight on down, Rory will be waiting for you,' she almost smirked down the phone. She bounded over from the front desk and told me with a beaming smile on her face that there was a puppy on the way that was bleeding from his mouth, and she would be ready and waiting in the pub once I was finished. Unfortunately, as it turned out, in her delight at having an emergency call, she had forgotten to take any details from the owner so the only information she could give me was that they sounded very upset and concerned about their young puppy. When dealing with an emergency, information is key. For example, in this case, I could have been dealing with anything from a collapsed puppy gasping for breath, bleeding from its lungs, to a puppy that had gone and played with a lawn mower. Thankfully it turned out to be nothing that serious.

Either way, I had to prepare for all possibilities, so I spent the next fifteen minutes with the nurse, prepping and checking the emergency drugs, setting up the oxygen supply, materials for an intravenous catheter and the fluids for managing blood loss and shock. There is something about the time you spend waiting for an emergency – it is almost as if time slows down and you end up going over things in your head again and again. It's an odd feeling, but it's almost like the whole team becomes a coiled spring ready to burst into action, like a field of sprinters poised and ready to go upon hearing the start gun.

Despite her suggestion of waiting in the pub, the receptionist was still there when the puppy came in. She whipped the dog off the concerned owner as they came bursting into the clinic, and brought it straight through to the nurse and me, waiting in the prep area. This is generally the best approach with these sorts of cases: urgency is key. The few minutes it can take to see the owner in and admit them through a consult room, instead of just taking the animal and rushing it straight through to where you have set up your emergency gear, can make the difference between life and death.

I was waiting by the prep table when the receptionist came running through the door, puppy in her arms. I scooped the little guy off her and popped him on the table. He had a little bit of blood staining around his mouth and a little on his front right paw. He sat there and looked at me, then he cocked his head to the side as if to ask, 'Why am I here, human? What's all the fuss about?' He was a gorgeous little Staffie, couldn't have been more than six months old, with a deep blue coat with the sheen you only see in puppies. He stood up on all fours and started to wag his tail in a playful manner. His tail was like a whip moving from side to side and had a weird, circular motion that meant as he wagged it, his whole body seemed to wag with it. That, paired with his open-mouth grin, made him an absolute heart-melter.

I carried on with my exam, starting to think that maybe we weren't going to need all the kit we had set up. I listened to his chest – 'heart rate one-twenty, chest clear,' I reported to my nurse as she scribbled on a piece of paper. 'Abdomen soft and comfy, no fluid thrill, temperature normal,' I continued. I finished my head-to-tail exam and then went to open his mouth and, as I did this, he let out a yelp as one of his canine teeth came out into my palm. He yawned at me, allowing me a really good look at his little puppy teeth being pushed from beneath the gum line by a new set of adult gnashers. I smiled to myself as he started licking my nose, his puppy breath rich and slightly tinged with the iron-y smell of blood. I don't know about you, but I love puppy breath!

I walked back through to the waiting area with the puppy under my arm. The client stood up as soon as he saw me coming, almost throwing the cup of tea the receptionist had made him all over the freshly mopped floor. He ran up to me and grabbed the puppy, his concerned look almost turning to annoyance when he saw me smiling.

'Nothing to worry about Mr Williams, this little guy is just teething,' I said.

'He's knocked a tooth out?' the owner replied in horror.

'Yes,' I said, 'but that's completely normal. It's because his adult teeth are coming through.'

'What do you mean?' he asked.

'Well, you know how children lose their baby teeth when they're young? Puppies do the same,' I explained to the clearly confused client.

'Oh wow, I didn't realise puppies did that,' he replied, his expression softening as he started to realise his puppy wasn't in danger. 'Thank God, this was the first night my girlfriend has let me look after Bruno on my own and I thought I had broken him,' he laughed. We exchanged a bit of friendly chat as he finished his cup of tea. He thanked me for my time and I jokingly thanked him for letting me get away on time. The first time I had left on time that week, I later realised.

*

It's amazing how few people realise other animals can lose their baby teeth. I must get this kind of confusion at least once a month, so I have started warning new puppy owners. It's a funny one, seeing their reactions when I explain that between four and six months of age their puppies will go from having 28 sharp little needles to 42 pearly whites. Some look at me like I'm an idiot, clearly thinking I'm talking rubbish, while others are quite shocked. I once had a little girl come to see me with her puppy and proudly exclaim that he had lost a tooth, which she had dutifully cleaned and put under her pillow for the tooth fairy. To her surprise, the tooth fairy hadn't left her a £5 note like normal (kids these days. I used to get 20p!), but in its place a bag of puppy treats. I looked at the mum and she just shrugged as if to say, 'What was I meant to do?'

As the owner left with his beautiful little Staffie pup, I looked at the smug receptionist. She had a grin from ear to ear. I weighed up trying to argue the validity of a baby tooth being a true emergency but thought better of it and just accepted that she had been right. I grabbed my things and we headed to the pub.

Going to the pub after a shift is something I do regularly. When you work in a job that is so demanding, it is important to wind down. I have also always believed that you should socialise with the people you work with – working with people you call friends is way more fun than those that you call colleagues. When I was a student, I was always invited to the pub with the vets and nurses where I was seeing practice. I was so happy to be included and it really taught me the importance of socialising with your colleagues outside of work.

It's funny to think back to being a student: spending time in a busy practice quickly becomes second nature. It's part of the professional training I guess, spending hours and hours shadowing, observing day-to-day life. Not only do you get to familiarise yourself with the quirks of every day veterinary life (such as Friday night emergencies), but you also learn an incredible amount. Any vets or vet students reading this will know that feeling, getting home after a day of being a student in practice; to this day I don't think I've known tiredness like it, before or since. As a student you're constantly being hit with questions or jobs, all the while panicking because putting one foot wrong might make you look incompetent. You have spent the last three years in lectures and reading in the library (haven't you?), preparing to be the best vet you can be. Then once you're on placement, you're in full view to be judged by your future colleagues, as worthy or not worthy of the profession you have dreamt of for years. Don't mess it up . . . Well, here's a little piece of advice to anyone out there who is going through vet training or anything similar: everyone makes mistakes, everyone has done stupid shit, everyone hits bumps in the road. Learn from it and then move on – you'll definitely be a better vet for it.

*

As I have mentioned, I have wanted to be a vet since I was a very young boy. There were times when I weighed up vet versus doctor, and at moments (and I mean very brief moments) of complete insanity, accountant, but becoming a vet was always a pretty easy winner. All things medical have always fascinated me. Before getting into veterinary school and starting my training, my sister and I used to spend hours on end watching medical TV shows. *Scrubs* was our favourite. I always dreamt about trying to be the real-life 'JD' of the veterinary world. Then I started at uni and *House* was my thing. I'm sure anyone who has ever had to revise has factored in revision breaks, and episodes of *House* with carrots and hummus was my break of choice during second-year exams.

When people think of vets, I suspect the big hospital with the hundreds of specialists doing high-tech, life-saving work probably isn't quite what they imagine. I know that until I reached university I envisaged the mixed-practice style of veterinary – driving around the countryside in an old banger, full to the brim with all sorts of medical gear that could have been produced in the 1920s and being called out at three o'clock in the morning to deliver a dairy calf. Doesn't it sound wonderful? But places like the Queen Mother Hospital at the Royal Veterinary College and other big hospitals around the country (and the world) are doing incredible, world-leading surgery and medicine day in, day out. Things that you haven't even conceived for an animal are now possible these days due to dedicated specialists, who take human medical techniques and innovations and push the boundaries of modern-day veterinary. I must admit, when I was studying, it was that world I wanted to be a part of. I wanted to be the veterinary version of Dr House and perform life-saving procedures and diagnose incredibly rare diseases day in, day out. Alas, that has not happened, but a boy could dream.

As well as wanting to be a super-duper specialist, I had a particular penchant for emergency work. In your final year and a half of training you start to get really stuck in to real-life vet work on what they call 'rotations'. This essentially consists of spending a week or two with each service in the hospital, training in the most advanced levels of care available to our pets. 'Services' in the hospital include, but are not limited to, anaesthesia, cardiology, dermatology, diagnostic imaging, emergency medicine, internal medicine, neurology, oncology, ophthalmology ... you get the gist. While on these rotations, depending which service you were with and, more importantly, which clinician you had to answer to, the work load could vary hugely.

I will never forget my anaesthesia rotation. The rotation was renowned among the students as the hardest of the lot. It was one of the 'on-call' rotations, meaning as well as working five days a week, you had to cover a weekend *and* possibly be called in overnight if you were the unlucky student on call when a poorly animal had to be rushed into theatre. There was one particular clinician who was feared by the students. There are always wonderfully exaggerated stories of these characters and the stories about him did not disappoint.

'I heard he once made a student stand in front of a white board for eight hours staring at a diagram of a dog's lungs because they didn't know the blood supply!'

'That's nothing. I heard he made a student put IV catheters into their own arm for practice because they couldn't get one on their patient!'

'Well, I heard he fails one student every week just for fun.'

For the purpose of this story he shall be 'Mr A'. You know, like Mr Anaesthesia.

*

I turned up for my first day on anaesthesia in a bit of a state. I had been in the USA for the preceding four weeks carrying out an externship in Florida. It was my final year of vet school and I was loving it. At last the years of intricate study of physiology and anatomy of animals were paying off and I was allowed to get hands-on with animals.

It was what I had always dreamt vet school to be. I had been staying with my aunt and uncle in their massive Floridian home, the weather had been somewhere in the region of 30°C every day and, for some unknown reason, my aunt had trusted me to drive her sports car. Yeah, I had had a pretty good time. Four weeks in a veterinary surgery in the USA had got me thinking about heading out there to work. I loved the hospital: it was open, spacious and the staff were super friendly (in that American way). I hadn't really prepared for it but word got round by my second or third week, and people were coming in to see 'the British doctor'. Despite me regularly telling the customers that I really wasn't a 'doctor' and they most definitely did not want me seeing their animals, I ended up running my own clinics, overseen by the head vet. The thing I loved about working in the USA (no, it wasn't being 'the British doctor') was the variety of species you would see in a week. Because of the diversity of the wildlife out there, we regularly had to treat crocs, incredibly colourful species of bird and, most commonly, turtles and terrapins. Because Florida is a wetland area with huge lakes the size of small oceans, there is a lot of water life around.

Turtles are a hugely common finding and this was super exciting for an animal lover like me; there is nothing quite like seeing animals in their natural habitat. Unfortunately, due to increasing human intervention, the number of lakes in the area is getting smaller and so the local wildlife are getting confused and confined. I was really taken aback when I was handed my first turtle: they can be pretty big animals and this one was a bit of a monster. He had a very small crack in his shell that I was told to 'patch up'. What do you patch up a turtle's shell with? I hear you ask ... epoxy resin. Yup, that's right. In my time at the clinic in Florida, I became a bit of a dab hand at fixing these amazing animals up. Roads are a huge threat to the local wildlife, especially during mating season when the males will often try to cross the road to find a mate. It isn't uncommon to see dead turtles on the side of the road, but the local vets help with what they can. In the UK I had always had a love for wildlife. At the wildlife centre I had worked at in the Cotswolds as a teenager I had helped treat injured hedgehogs, foxes, badgers, deer, birds and more; they were all incredible creatures but I hadn't dealt with anything quite like a turtle before. I was just about getting used to the scaly beasts by week three in Florida – one had even decided to try and take a chunk out of my hand while I wasn't looking.

'You never really and truly know an animal until they give you a nip,' one of the vets had said, laughing, as I dripped blood from my hand. Turns out turtle beaks can pack a real punch.

'You won't want a bite from the next wild animal you see. Come find me in about a half hour,' she said, still chuckling to herself at my misfortune. I patched myself up and went off for lunch and then, as she had asked, I went off to find her. After trawling the clinic, I eventually found her in the car park with her head in the back of a pickup truck. I headed over and when I saw what she was examining I stopped in my tracks. There was a big wildcat lying in the back of the pickup, sedated, with the vet pulling its back leg around, examining it. It was a cougar, a Labrador-sized cat. The vet was correct: I definitely didn't want to get acquainted with that bite!

*

The days were long and it had been hard work, but I loved every minute of being in Florida. All until the journey home. I had booked a flight to get me back to the UK on the Sunday morning, knowing I had anaesthesia to deal with the day after. I boarded the plane at Tampa, a quick hop to Miami and then a direct flight back to the UK. Easy.

Oh, how wrong I was. We sat on the runway at Tampa, as I watched the minute hand on my watch. I had planned for fifty minutes' transfer time at Miami airport which, yes, was probably cutting it a touch fine, and after thirty minutes still on the tarmac in Florida, it was looking unlikely that I would make my flight to London.

We took off, the seatbelt signs went off and I pushed the 'call' button above my seat. I must admit, before this flight I had never pressed it and almost felt like a naughty child doing so now. As a kid, I used to have to press every button I physically could. Honestly, even to this day I can't get in a new car without fiddling with all the buttons and dials.

The flight attendant came over. 'Hello sir, how can I help you today?' She was quite possibly the most American woman I had ever encountered.

'Well, um, I was just thinking, I have a transfer flight to London from Miami and as we are running half an hour behind I am a touch concerned that I may, well, miss it. Is there any way of knowing if I'll make it?' I bumbled through my sentence, trying not to get distracted by her blonde locks and bright red lipstick.

She smiled sweetly, the same smile I had received from most women in Florida when I opened my mouth and my terrible, clumsy, overly posh English accent escaped into the world (I'm sure I became more English when I went over there!). 'Oh, I'm sure we can get you onto that flight. The pilot thinks we are going to make up a heap of time. I'll keep checking back on you with updates, honey.'

I just smiled back at her. I must have looked completely gormless, and I felt it too. I spent the flight with one eye on my watch, the other trying to read through the BSAVA guide to small animal anaesthesia.

We touched down at Miami and I had exactly twenty-four minutes to get from my gate to where the Airbus A380 was waiting to fly me home. I got to my gate with just six minutes to spare. I was going to get home in time for my rotation. I wasn't going to become another victim of Mr A, made to recite all fifty states of America in alphabetical order before being allowed back on campus (or something equally absurd).

There was one slight hiccup. I may have made the plane and got back to London as hoped, but guess what? My bag didn't. Not just my suitcase with all my clothes, but also the suitcase with my medical textbooks, my stethoscope, my scrub tops and every nice pair of trousers and shirts I owned (which wasn't many – I was a student after all). I got home and tried to work out how to play it. There was only really one option and that was to succumb to my fate.

I rocked up on Monday morning to my first day of my anaesthesia rotation. I had not done the suggested reading for the week as my books were in the suitcase. I was wearing a ten-year-old shirt that did that weird parting thing a shirt does around your chest when it is too small. I had no scrub top to cover my shirt; I didn't have a stethoscope, thermometer or any other part of the expected kit a veterinary student should carry, as they were all tucked away neatly in my suitcase. I was also five minutes late and very jet lagged which, I'm sure when you're teaching at a veterinary hospital and used to dealing with students, no doubt looks less like jet lag and a lot more like a hangover. I was fucked.

As I ran from the bus stop across to the hospital I said a little prayer to myself that we had lucked out as a group and got a nice clinician. There was a whole plethora of lovely anaesthesia residents and clinicians – not least 'Team Spain'. There are certain disciplines in veterinary that seem to appeal to Spanish and Italian vets. I don't know why, but it always seemed that they came in groups, hence the students terming the three Spanish anaesthesia residents 'Team Spain'. They were really lovely. Maybe we would get one of them, I prayed as I ran. I arrived at the hospital and slowed to a fast walk. Unless there was a crash alarm sounding, there was a 'no running' policy in the hospital to save anyone going arse over tit when careering into a Labrador on a hospital trolley. I sped through the corridor to the anaesthesia room and took a deep breath before pushing through the swing doors. I must have looked like I had been dragged through a hedge backwards – the faces of my classmates certainly suggested so, ranging from disgust to mild amusement. I snuck to the back of my colleagues like a scorned puppy, my face not just flushed from rushing through the hospital, but now turning a nice shade of beetroot at the embarrassment of being such a mess on day one. I had bundled into the room just as Mr A was giving his welcome speech and introduction to the anaesthesia rotation. I thought I had got away with it. I had just about returned to a normal human colour as the briefing came to an end and, with horror, I saw Mr A make a beeline for me.

'Any particular reason you were late to my briefing . . .' he looked down at my shirt, looking for my name-embossed scrub top, 'and why are you not wearing your scrub top?'

'I'm really sorry Mr A, it's a very long story – my bag got left in Miami and all my things are in it . . .' I started at a rate of knots.

He looked at me as if to say 'you think I'm going to buy that shit?'

I stopped. 'I'm sorry Mr A, I will have my things tomorrow. Is there a spare top I can put on for today?' He smirked and assured me he would find one. Mr A seemed to take a liking to me after that day. Whenever he needed something doing for the following two weeks he would shout my name and inevitably, like a good whipping boy, I would be there to help. By no means was this due to my incredible veterinary knowledge or my promising future as an anaesthesia intern. Nope, I'm pretty sure it was because Mr A had a very tiny, almost nonexistent but definitely there, modicum of respect for me. I had, after all, spent the first day of the rotation wearing the top he had kindly found me. The extra small, neon pink scrub top.

*

As much as I enjoyed my anaesthesia rotation, the one I relished even more was emergency medicine. This entailed working days, nights and weekends to keep the most critical and unwell of patients alive and treating the weirdest, and most wonderful, of conditions. The work really appealed to the problem-solver in me and, being a bit of an adrenaline junkie, it was right up my street. It was in the emergency room I felt most at home, running blood gas analysis, helping with advanced ventilator cases, dealing with traumas and helping out in crash calls. There is nothing quite like the rush you get from saving a life.

5

Into the Lion's Den

It should come as no real surprise then when I tell you that my first job was in a twenty-four hour hospital and I was very quickly on shift work. I worked a rolling rota of four days on, four days off, four nights on, four days off. It was a dream to be working in such a busy hospital and I loved every minute of it, almost. My first day, however, was also the first day I cried as a vet too.

Five years of training, seeing practice, endless hours of lectures, working on farms and gruelling exams had all led to this. I was finally a vet. I had secured myself a job offer a few weeks before I sat finals, a risky strategy as it piled on more pressure to pass those exams. But I got through it and graduated, with my first day at my first job looming. I spent an initial few weeks seeing the practice, in and out of branch work and shadowing my mentors to get to grips with real-life vetting, before being let loose on shift work.

Veterinary is a bit like driving. When you learn to drive, you spend months behind the wheel, learning to check that blind spot, when to signal, how to hill start and make a three-point turn, but when you actually pass your driving test it's a completely different experience. You spend the following months learning how to really drive, like an actual human being, not a robot.

Veterinary is kind of the same. You come out of vet school having spent five years learning everything from the basic functions of the canine digestive tract to the stay-apparatus of the horse (the incredible anatomical feature that horses possess, allowing them to lock their legs out to support their massive weight), and suddenly you have to be hands-on with your own real-life patients and their owners. What's more, you have to put on a decent enough act of knowing what you're doing, so that, number one, you don't kill the patient, and number two, you convince the owner that you deserve to be in that consult room. Don't get me wrong, young vets know all they need to – hell, some of the students I work with these days know incredible amounts of detail that I could only have dreamt of retaining after vet school. But there is always that question when you're a young vet. The worry that you aren't as good as the more experienced vets and the owner is going to catch you out. That the demon sat on your shoulder, whispering in your ear, telling you that you aren't good enough, is actually right.

The beauty of hindsight and knowledge allows me to look back on this and identify it as textbook 'imposter syndrome'. Imposter syndrome is something I struggled with from day one: the feeling of inadequacy. I was constantly worried that I wasn't as good as my colleagues. I don't know where the insecurity comes from but it was there right from the start.

Even nowadays I sometimes have to remind myself that I am good at what I do. Imposter syndrome is defined as 'a psychological pattern in which one doubts one's accomplishments and has a persistent, internalised fear of being exposed as a "fraud" despite external evidence of their competence. Individuals with impostor syndrome attribute their success to luck, or interpret it as a result of deceiving others into thinking they are more intelligent than they perceive themselves to be.' When I first read that definition it was like someone had reached into my psyche and placed it on a piece of paper.

My first 'real' day was a twelve-hour shift at the main hospital. It was a massive, grey building just south of London and my first taste of South London suburbia. I had been there a few times before, but on this particular day it felt more daunting than ever. At the time I was living in Lewisham. I was renting my first flat on my own, and I felt so grown up. I spent my first commute into work wondering what I might end up seeing or doing on my first real day's work. I kept getting pangs of mild panic as my mind wandered to complex medical diagnoses and angry owners. After all, I had always had a bit of a safety blanket up until now.

As a student I had been lucky to be trusted by the vet I was shadowing with my own list of consults, so I felt that I had a bit of a head start on other newly graduated vets, having had first-hand experience of dealing with the public and their animals. Saying that, even then, I had always had a senior, experienced vet in the next room to run to if I felt out of my comfort zone or, worse, did something stupid.

I was sitting in my car on the South Circular at seven o'clock in the morning, my stomach in knots; it was all getting a bit real. I eventually managed to park my 2010 Ford Fiesta right next to what I assumed was the boss's new Jaguar. I caught myself thinking it must have cost him a bob or two, and was immediately ashamed of myself for thinking exactly what a client would have thought at the sight of the shiny new car. I wandered in and started my twelve-hour shift.

From the word go, I had four patients under my care. I had taken a handover from the night vet, a young guy from New Zealand who, to me, was king of emergency medicine. He was an incredible vet: fast acting, always had the answers, exactly what you wanted from a night vet. He had had a bit of a killer night, which had included a cat that had been hit by a car, a diabetic that had gone into a hypoglycaemic crisis, a dog that had eaten a whole box of raisins (which, despite me regularly sharing mine with my dog as a child, can cause acute and fatal kidney disease in dogs), box and all, and most recently a Boxer dog called Ralph.

Ralph had come in about twenty minutes before I started my shift. I had seen his owners leaving as I walked through the car park. I had assumed they were mother and daughter, the mother a squat woman in a green parka with a fur hood. She had a terribly friendly face, the face of a woman who would have taken one look at me and immediately made me a sandwich 'to put some meat on your bones', but as I walked past her in the car park, tears were dripping from her chin. The daughter was much taller and slimmer, probably early thirties, and had her arm around her, consoling. I just heard a small part of what she was muttering to her mother: 'It's okay, Mum, he will be home in a few days, I promise . . .'

I sprang up the stairs to the staff room, dropped my stuff and changed into my scrubs. The way the hospital worked was that if you were a consulting vet, i.e. you spent your day in consults seeing animals for anything from vaccinations to chronic illnesses you can hardly pronounce and you wore an ironed (I never ironed mine, to the outrage of my boss), blue-and-white-striped, short-sleeve shirt. Yeah, they were gross. The reason I never ironed mine was in protest at the short-sleeve nature of the shirts. Short sleeve makes a lot of sense in a medical setting with 'bare below the elbow' being something that is hammered into you at university, but come on . . . a short-sleeve, button-up shirt?! Anyway, that didn't matter on my first day as I was on a hospital shift, and when you worked that shift, you were in full scrubs. They were dark blue and I felt so unbelievably cool, like a doctor off the television – maybe I was finally going to be a real-life 'Dr House'.

I checked myself in the mirror, ran my hand through my hair and gave myself a light slap on the cheeks. 'You got this,' I reassured myself, and I headed downstairs to the prep room.

The 'prep room' is the heart of any veterinary practice which ties everything together. If you have ever been to a vet's, they may have suggested taking your pet 'to the back' or 'to the prep room' for some bloods or some other tests. The basic building blocks of a veterinary practice are the reception, the consult room, the pharmacy, the prep room, the imaging suite or X-ray room, depending on how big the practice is, the surgical theatre, possibly a dental suite although often this is just a tub-table in the prep room, and then the wards. Again, depending on the practice, you may have one ward, you may have specific dog and cat wards, or you may even be lucky enough to have an exotic pet ward as well. Only in the really big referral hospitals will you have a ward for all different types of patients as in a human hospital, for example a cardiology ward, a neurology ward and a separate medical and surgical ward. Any patient that is having any sort of procedure or investigation done will likely be in the prep room, either for the entirety or at least the majority of their time while being looked at by the vets or nurses. Indeed, the prep room is where I found Kevin the night vet with Ralph on that first morning.

Ralph was a four-year-old Boxer dog that had come in to see my new colleague at ten past seven. The reason for his trip to the vet was frequent, aggressive seizures that had been happening for just over two hours. His owner, Cheryl, had struggled to get him into the vet's despite knowing he needed to be seen urgently, because she was sixty-four years old and picking up a thirty-something kilogram Boxer dog while it paddled uncontrollably was no mean feat. The two hours she took to get him to the vet were mainly filled with panicked phone calls to her daughter and her husband, asking them to come over with their 4x4 so they could get him to see a vet as soon as possible.

Kevin had met them in the car park, something I would do for dozens of emergencies over the coming eighteen months, and had scooped Ralph up and run him through to the prep area, undoubtedly making the heavy dog look like a mere Chihuahua. Yeah, Kevin worked out. He had swiftly placed an intravenous catheter into Ralph's cephalic vein (the most commonly used vein for intravenous access in dogs, found in the front leg), and taken some blood from his jugular vein (the most commonly used vein for blood taking, found either side of the neck). Whenever dealing with a seizuring dog, the first thing to do after they stop seizuring is to check organ function and look for any signs of toxicity. This starts to give you a bit of an idea as to why the dog is seizuring and why their brain is essentially trying to fry itself. The list of possible causes for a seizuring dog includes the ingestion of toxins, such as chewing gum, brain tumours, liver disease, trauma, epilepsy and a number of other diseases.

Ralph's bloods were taken upstairs where one of the lab technicians started urgently running them through the high-tech machines. The lab techs were some of my favourite people in the hospital from day one. They were called Jane and Sarah, were both middle-aged and had worked at the hospital for a number of years. On my first tour of the practice, while everyone else seemed a little busy to say hello to the new guy, they had been there with beaming smiles and offering wide open arms for a big hug. By the time I started my first hospital shift, I had already adopted them as my practice 'mums' and they were always my go-to for a quiet chat and a cuppa. That being said, when it came down to business, they were a well-oiled machine, setting centrifuges whirring and lab machines buzzing at a rate of knots and delivering any number of lab results in a matter of moments.

Unfortunately or fortunately for Ralph (I was unsure at that point), there was no sign of any problems on his blood panel. He had beautiful organ function, as you would expect from a four-year-old dog, and we were no closer to an explanation for his seizuring. It was as the blood results came through that I was officially handed Ralph as my case. Kevin had started the diagnostics and my task was to keep him stabilised and stop him from seizuring for the next twelve hours – easy, right? The eventual plan was, if we could manage to stop him seizuring, to get him referred to a neurologist for an MRI scan – if Cheryl could afford it, that is. Kevin had given some emergency treatment to stop the seizuring: diazepam administered as an injection into the vein. It had worked beautifully: Ralph was no longer convulsing.

I stood there and looked at my patient. He was a big Boxer dog, lying flat on his side on the floor, too big for the conventional examination table which his legs would have poked over the edge of. I remember looking from his head to his tail, his chest rising and falling heavily as he sucked oxygen in, trying to fight the sedative effect of the anti-epilepsy drug he had just been given. Not only was this my first real medical patient, the first time I had been handed over a case, my first time in the hospital on a 'proper' shift, but it was also the first time I felt that utter and all-consuming fear that would become my constant companion for the next few weeks (or months if you want the truth). I was Ralph's only hope here; his life was quite literally, and ever so scarily, in my hands for the next twelve hours.

Ralph, at that point, was stable. The drugs had worked, and he was sedated and not seizuring. His blood had come back normal so for now it was a case of wait and see. That gave me time to head round the hospital and see my other three patients . . . yeah, remember those other animals I mentioned?

Firstly, the cat that had thought it a good idea to play chicken with a speeding BMW. As you can imagine, it didn't go terribly well for Fluffy. Cats are well known for their speed and smarts but poor old Fluffy wasn't the cleverest cookie. She had started to cross the road, taken seat and started licking her arse as the BMW careered towards her. Quite luckily, although also rather distressingly, the owner had happened to look out of the window at the exact moment that Fluffy realised there was a car behind her and managed a backwards cartwheel out of the way. She almost got away with it too, had she not left her right back leg trailing for the car's front bumper to crack as it sped on past. Of course the driver didn't stop, and, as the law stipulates, that is technically legal as long as it wasn't intended animal cruelty.

As a side note, if it had been a dog the car hit, the driver would legally need to stop and try to find the owner to report the 'criminal damage' they just caused. The British legal system, ladies and gentlemen . . .

That right back leg, unfortunately for poor old Fluffy, was now bandaged up in a big cast ready for me to X-ray later that day. I popped into the kennel and gave her a bit of fuss, and she purred and rolled over for a belly rub; that's what I love about cats – they can have multiple fractures in their right hind limb but as long as they get the good pain drugs, they bloomin' love a fuss (mostly).

Next was Simba – a distinguished old gentleman cat who had been diagnosed with diabetes years ago. Diabetes is when the body cannot control how much sugar is in the blood. In humans there are two types of diabetes: type one and type two. In cats, it is thought that they get something similar to type two. To control diabetes in cats, you more often than not have to inject them with insulin twice a day. This sounds scary and can be really daunting for owners at first, but Simba's owners had taken to this like ducks to water, and were now absolute pros. The day before Simba found himself in hospital with me, Simba's dad was starting a new job and got up an hour earlier than usual. He had treated it like any other morning: get up, shower, shave, feed Simba, have breakfast, inject Simba's insulin, head off to work. This was absolutely spot on, a perfectly rehearsed routine. What made Simba's day go from rather peachy to pretty rubbish was when his mum got up and decided that his dad couldn't possibly have given Simba his insulin with his new super early routine, so she repeated the injection. A few hours later and Simba was lying on the floor unable to lift his head and in need of an emergency trip to the vet's. The good news was that Kevin had sorted this out with a glucose drip and Simba, just like little Fluffy, was feeling much better, and if he stayed well could go home that afternoon. 'Thankfully,' I thought, while reviewing Simba's chart, 'there isn't much for me to do with Simba. More time for Ralph.'

Thirdly, we had Bruce. When you hear the name Bruce, you think Bulldog, you think Staffie, you do not think Pomeranian . . . Well, that's exactly what Bruce was, a 3kg Pomeranian with a personality quite reminiscent of what I imagine Attila the Hun's was. Little Bruce lived with a couple and their young daughter. Like any good parents, the owners had been battling to try to get their daughter to eat more fruit and vegetables, which as I'm sure some of you can relate to, can be a tricky business.

It so happened that Bruce and the little girl were best of friends – they were inseparable. Incredibly, the owners had chanced upon a bit of a trick when the dad had dropped a carrot on the floor one Sunday that Bruce quickly snaffled.

From that day on, the daughter ate carrots. If it was good enough for Bruce, it was good enough for her. They had therefore spent the last few weeks feeding Bruce different vegetables and fruits to get their daughter to eat them, with unbelievable success.

Yesterday, however, the dad had tried raisins, and not just one raisin, a whole packet, which, as he was later told by his wife, can be severely toxic to some dogs. Cue three days at the vet's on an IV drip for little Bruce. Ordinarily this is a bit of a nightmare, let alone when Bruce decides that no-one is allowed to touch him at pain of a very nasty bite. I must admit, it always seems to be the difficult animals that end up spending the longest time in hospital. I glanced through the bars as he looked up from his sleep, one eye watching my every move. He was doing well (I ascertained from a safe distance) and I returned to Ralph.

I walked up to the gorgeous Boxer dog. He was lying on a thick bed, covered by a blanket. As I approached, he looked up at me with sad eyes that hurt me right in my heart. He was asking for help, confused and scared about where he was and what was going on.

Something I will never become immune to is the look of helplessness a dog can give. It shakes me to my core and drives an eternal need to help in me that nothing else even comes close to. As he looked at me, I thought I saw his eyes twitch from side to side. They settled but then I was sure I saw it happen a second time. I knelt down beside him just as his eyes flickered again, more violently this time, and then he started full blown seizuring. It was violent: his jaws clamped shut, his neck muscles tensed, throwing his head back, his legs became rigid, sticking straight out, and then he started convulsing, his legs paddled and his whole body shook. It was like he was possessed, his sad expression of a few moments before most definitely gone and replaced by a demon-like presence. I was taken aback; I had never seen a dog seizure before in real life, only in videos, and it was truly terrifying. The only way to describe it is like something had taken over Ralph's body and he had lost all control.

I just stood there watching, feet rooted to the floor, not really sure of what to do. One of the senior nurses was a few metres behind me, and heard the commotion as Ralph started scrabbling against the walls.

Like a coiled spring she jumped past me, pushing me to the side, seeing that I was clearly going to be of little use. She grabbed a pre-loaded diazepam injection that Kevin had left out for just this sort of thing, and injected the contents into Ralph's intravenous line. After a few seconds, it was as if the demon left his body. He stopped trying to run in mid-air, his eyes came forwards from the back of his head and his whole body relaxed; he was back in the room. I had been useless, just stood there like a lemon while my only really critical patient was having a hugely violent fit. The nurse got up from Ralph's side and put a hand on my shoulder, clearly able to see I was shell-shocked. 'It's okay, that's a tough first case you've got there. Draw up some more emergency drugs and keep a close eye. If he does it again, just give him a dose and repeat if necessary. You'll be fine,' she said.

So I did exactly that. I replaced the diazepam and sat down on the floor next to Ralph. He was pretty out of it with the drugs he had been given, but whenever I moved or muttered anything his tail went like a paddle. I thought to myself what a wonderful dog he must be and made a promise under my breath that I would make him better.

Ten minutes later, we were just settling into a comfy spot in the kennel when he seizured again, and this time I was on it. I grabbed for the drugs and gave them within about ten seconds. I sat and watched, waiting for him to come out of the seizure. He didn't. Thirty seconds passed and he was still going, paddling like he was trying to run along the wall. He wasn't going to come out of this one – it was too severe. I gave him another dose of anti-epileptic drugs and still he just carried on going. He seizured for a full three minutes, which I knew because I had clocked the time on my phone as he had started. There wasn't much to do other than let him come out of it, but this was really not good.

Once he was out of the episode, I leant down, reassured him and went to call his mum. The phone rang and rang but no answer came, so I left a message for Cheryl, or Mrs Johns as I had addressed her, to call me as soon as she could. We needed a plan.

As I went back to the ward, a little dejected and worried that I hadn't manage to speak to Ralph's owner to keep her in the loop, I could tell something was wrong. Ralph was seizuring again and it could only have been about fifteen minutes since the last one. This was not good at all. I darted into the ward and the nurses explained that they had given two more doses of diazepam but there was no response. There was only one option left.

I turned and ran across the room to the drugs cupboard. I grabbed a bottle labelled Propofol and ran back to Ralph. The only option now was to put Ralph under anaesthetic to stop the seizures. I injected the cloudy white liquid into him and the seizuring stopped. Unlike the last time, though, his body just went limp. I placed an endotracheal tube into the back of his throat so that we could control his breathing and deliver oxygen. By this point I had a team of amazing nurses around me all helping in any way they could. I left Ralph in their capable hands and went to work out another dose of Propofol for him.

My plan was to keep Ralph on a continuous injection of the white liquid to keep him asleep for a few hours to allow his brain to cool down and his body to relax. We would keep him on this constant rate infusion (known as a CRI in the vet world) for a few hours, and then slowly wean him off until he became conscious, and hopefully, seizure-free. That was the aim.

The problem with ongoing regular and violent seizures is that the brain starts to heat up. It is full of temperature sensitive tissues and enzymes that, if the environment gets too hot, stop working. In severe cases this can cause lasting brain damage and in the worst cases, death.

Ralph was stable for now, with a nurse sitting next to him, keeping a close eye. My other patients were all okay, either awaiting procedures or being looked after by other vets. I looked down at my watch: it was coming up for eleven o'clock. 'Wow,' I thought to myself, 'how time flies when you're running around like a headless chicken.' I felt almost guilty, but I went and got a cup of coffee and found a corner to sit and read up on neurology in dogs, waiting for Cheryl to call me back.

At the hospital we were lucky to have a large collection of books as reference for almost any case we had. In my time there I occasionally found myself fishing out a random textbook to fill the time on dragging night shifts. I've always found that it's the obscure things that fascinate me, so despite being a pet vet, I was often drawn to the exotic animal books, regularly settling on *Fowler's Zoo* and *Wild Animal Medicine*. I'm still waiting to astound colleagues with my secret knowledge of giraffe medicine. On that day, though, it was a canine neurology textbook.

I always get a pang of guilt when opening a textbook to research a condition or disease of a patient of mine. There is a part of me that expects my brain to be able to retain knowledge about every condition of every species, with every diagnostic test and treatment protocol, which of course is impossible. During my training, there was a medicine professor who was regarded as an encyclopaedia of knowledge; he could tell you the most obscure detail about the rarest of diseases. He was also, incidentally, well known amongst students for performing a rectal examination upon every single one of his patients. I asked him once about this and he simply replied, 'A rectal is an essential part of a thorough physical examination, Rory,' and walked off. Either way, even this veterinary RainMan could be found trawling through textbooks on occasion.

I don't know why I was reading through the textbook – I knew the approach to a seizuring dog and we had followed it to the tee. It was rare that you had to go as far as putting a dog on a CRI of Propofol. Of course it was going to happen on my first real day as a vet (and this was to be the first and also the only time I have ever had to do this for a seizuring patient – yes, Ralph was really, really unwell). I think I was just trying to reassure myself that I was doing everything right before speaking to Mrs Johns and telling her things were not looking too great.

I picked up the phone and dialled again. By this point I had put two and two together and come to the conclusion that she must have been the squat, friendly-looking lady I had seen in the car park that morning.

She picked up this time. 'Hello?' Her voice was already a bit shaky as if she had been crying.

'Hi Mrs Johns, this is Rory. I'm the vet looking after Ralph today.' We chatted for about fifteen minutes. I took her through what had happened that morning since Ralph had been admitted and explained that he was currently under a prolonged anaesthetic to control the seizuring. She had hardly said a word as I spoke, just the occasional 'okay' or 'I understand' between muffled sobs.

I never really knew how I would deal with upset clients – after all, this was my first experience of it. I would class myself as a man who is in touch with his emotions, so I always thought I would struggle with highly emotive situations. As I chatted away on the phone to the clearly very upset owner, I was a bit surprised at how little it was affecting me at the time.

I came to the end of my unintentional monologue and asked Mrs Johns if she understood the plan of action, and that there was unfortunately not a huge amount more we could do other than what we were already doing. She said she did and took a deep breath.

'I promise I am doing everything I can for him, Mrs Johns,' I said softly.

She replied, 'I know dear, give him a big kiss from me,' and then she was gone in a flash, probably trying to stifle another outburst of tears.

I put the phone back on the cradle and took stock. I was okay. I had been clear with the owner and showed I cared without blubbing down the phone. Rightly or wrongly, I was proud of myself. I went back down to the ward and continued working on my in-patients.

The majority of my day was spent with Ralph. I sat with him for hours and called Mrs Johns three more times through the day, keeping her as up to date as possible with what was going on with her four-legged friend.

Ralph had taken a little piece of my heart too, not only as my first patient but oh my goodness he was a lovely dog. We weaned him off the Propofol at about two in the afternoon, and he had come round slowly over about half an hour. He had his head in my lap and kept looking up at me as if to say we were now best mates. It was now closing in on three o'clock and so far he had not seizured – things were looking up!

I went and took a fifteen-minute lunch break with my neurology textbook, a cheese and pickle sandwich and a coffee. As I skipped back downstairs to the prep room and bounced through the door, I could tell immediately that something was wrong. I looked through the swinging door to the dog ward as one of the nurses went flying through and my heart dropped, all I could see were the team stood round four flailing legs. Ralph was seizuring again.

I called Mrs Johns for the fifth time that day. I had told her in our last call just half an hour previously that it was looking promising and he had been awake almost half an hour without seizuring. I must have sounded optimistic on the phone as Mrs J had even said 'Calm down dear, let's not get ahead of ourselves.' She had been right, and now I was calling her with a completely different tone, which she of course picked up on immediately. 'Hi Mrs Johns . . .' I started.

'He's seizuring again, isn't he?' she cut in. I clearly needed to work on hiding my emotion in my voice.

'Unfortunately so,' I said, 'and I'm afraid it was really violent.' She sighed again, as she had many times that day. I felt I was really getting to know her, which was odd, having never actually met her.

'Okay, well, what can we do?' she asked, suddenly very matter of fact. I was a little surprised but took her through the options.

'Well. We are running out of options here, but we can refer Ralph on to a neurologist to see if they can stabilise him but I would be worried about him travelling. Otherwise . . .' I trailed off. I had never discussed this with a real live owner before and I suddenly found I was lost for words. Luckily for me, Mrs Johns knew exactly what the other option was.

'Okay,' she said. 'What do you think we should do?' I settled the matter by suggesting that Mrs J came in to see me and Ralph and we speak face-to-face. This is something I still do to this day: no-one wants to have end-of-life conversations over the phone.

It was pushing four-thirty when the call came over the tannoy: 'Dr Rory to reception'. Mrs Johns had arrived. By this time, Ralph had had two more seizures and each one was sapping more and more energy from him. In-between the seizures he just lay on his side motionless, staring dead ahead almost pleading for some respite.

I went through to the reception area. It was a big hospital so, as you would imagine, there was a huge reception. On entering the hospital, the reception desk was in front of you with bright blue branding plastered all over the front of it. To the left of the desk you had the cat waiting area with hidey-holes for the cat baskets in an attempt to keep them more relaxed and stress-free. To the right of the desk, the dog waiting area with a wall of food and other bits for sale from doggy toothbrushes to the latest in fashionable dog coats. That is where I recognised Mrs Johns, sat huddled in her green parka, again with the taller younger woman who I had rightly assumed that morning was her daughter. I walked out and smiled at the pair. They got up and we convened in one of the consult rooms. I had decided to use the 'euthanasia room', not that it was publicised as that – that would have been a terrible way to break bad news. The room wasn't large, but not cramped, just very cosy, with a sofa and comfy chairs – not your average consulting room. Over the next eighteen months I was to become rather familiar with that room, and I must admit it was a nice touch to have a specific room for difficult conversations.

We sat and I offered them a cup of tea or coffee. They refused and got straight to the point: 'How is he? Can we see him?' I would have been the same.

'Absolutely, we can go and see him in a minute; I just want to have a chat first about where we are and what we can do.' The mother and daughter looked at each other.

'Well, we have discussed it and we just can't afford referral,' said Mrs Johns, 'I would do anything for him but it's just too much and I'm not sure it's fair on him.' I wasn't surprised by this – I had got a few quotes over the phone earlier that day and we were looking at least another thousand pounds to get him seen by a specialist, and that was without any guarantees that they would have any more success than we'd had. Mrs J had already expressed concerns over the cost to me earlier that day when I had told her what our bill would be.

'Okay, that's fine, that makes the decision more simple for us,' I started. 'We can carry on and give him more time, or . . .' I bowed my head – I just couldn't bring myself to say it. We all looked at each other in agreement. 'Okay, well, let me go and make sure he is ready for a visit and I'll be right back to get you.' I shuffled down the hall towards the dog kennel area, all the spring from earlier in the day completely gone from my step. I told the nurses that I was bringing the owners through and they all nodded solemnly. This wasn't standard practice, but I felt it was only fair as moving Ralph would likely cause him to seizure again.

I popped my head into his area: we had cleared the entire end of the ward for him so he could have a big plush bed with the lights off as to not rouse him, and a fan to cool his overheating body. He caught a glimpse of me and his long tail started to wag, beating the bed with a loud thump. I crept up to him gently and knelt by his head, 'Your mum is here, buddy,' I told him. 'You've gotta get better for her, okay?' He replied with a loud thump of his tail. I kissed him on the head and went back to the consult room. As the family caught a glimpse of Ralph they rushed towards him, but I grasped their arms as they started and reminded them to go slowly so as not to overexcite him. I could see it take every bit of self-control they had, but they listened and slowly approached their darling boy, whispering hellos as they went. They sat one each side of his head and I got a pillow for Mrs Johns as she had a bad hip but insisted she was going to sit down and cuddle him. I asked them if they needed anything and they said no. I left them to just be with their boy.

It was after five as I passed my boss in the hall as I was heading back to the staff room, 'How was day one, Rory? Finishing up?'

'No, I'm just with a patient and their family but I'm sure it won't be too long,' I lied and forced a smile. 'Day one has been tough,' I thought, but I kept that to myself. She muttered something cheery about not working too late and bumbled off on her way home. I walked through and sat in the vets' room – it was a tiny cubby hole, hardly big enough for four people despite the company employing over thirty vets. There were three computers for all to share, but at this time my colleagues were almost all either in consult or back at their respective branch practices for evening surgery. The main hospital was the hub of the veterinary clinic: it was massive and catered for all sorts of surgeries, with space for huge numbers of inpatients. The branch practices were dotted around as little satellites to allow the hospital to provide care for as big a number of animals as possible, often only staffed by a single vet and a receptionist. There was only one of my colleagues in the room tapping away at one of the computers and he turned to me as I wandered in, clearly seeing the weight of my day on my shoulders. It's weird, it's like there is a special 'vet code' that you only really understand once you're inducted into the profession. 'Tough first day, huh?' he commented.

'No, I'm all good, just a hard case – that's all.' I tried to shrug it off, but I could tell from his sideways glance that he knew I was talking out of my arse. He had had many days like this and I had many more to come. I was only starting to realise how taxing this job could be.

After about fifteen minutes, the tannoy rang out: 'Dr Rory to prep'. I pulled myself to my feet and went back to greet the Johns family. I crept into the dimly lit dog ward and sat beside the two women, Ralph in front of me. His head was resting on his mum's knee and all seemed peaceful, as if the world had come to a stand-still. I often think of that moment and it's odd, but every time I picture it I see it from another perspective. I see it as if I am standing at the end of the long dog ward, looking down towards the three of us and Ralph. We are silhouetted onto the back wall, four shadowed figures all sharing in the peace, draped in utter sorrow. Mrs Johns was slowly stroking Ralph's head and talking to him in a gentle whisper, telling him it was all going to be okay and not to worry himself one bit.

Once I had sat down, the daughter reached over and squeezed her mother's arm and then got up. 'I'm going to go and wait in the reception,' she said into mid-air, as if I wasn't there, and then left. People deal with death differently, some wanting to be with their animals and some, like Mrs Johns' daughter, not wanting to be there at all. I knew at that moment that they had come to the decision to put Ralph to sleep. I looked up at Mrs Johns as she continued to whisper softly to her darling boy – I didn't say anything and just sat there with her until she was ready. I held Ralph's paw and he reached out and put it on my lap, giving me a thud of his tail against his thick mattress bed. Even then there were still glimpses of the wonderful, happy dog Ralph was, despite what he was going through. Mrs Johns looked down at his paw in my hand and then up at me. She smiled through watery eyes and said, 'I think we have to say goodbye.' I placed my hand on hers and looked at her – I could see in her eyes how much Ralph meant to her and that her heart was breaking in front of me.

'Okay,' I replied simply and tried to find the facial expression between sad and understanding that I have spent years since trying to perfect.

We sat there for another ten minutes together, chatting about Ralph and what he had been like as a puppy, and we only stopped when a nurse came in with a clipboard and a syringe. Mrs Johns had been telling me a story about how Ralph once stole an entire Mr Whippy from a child in a pushchair but went silent as soon as she saw the door go, as if it was our secret. I handed her the form and asked her to read and sign it. Her hand was visibly shaking as she signed. 'Sorry,' she said, looking down at the wobbly scrawl she had left on the paper. I just smiled back.

We said our final goodbyes to Ralph, his tail still wagging at me as I finished injecting him. As he slipped away his whole body relaxed and a sense of calm came over him. Mrs Johns and I got up. I looked at her and she flung her arms around my neck. 'Thank you for everything, Rory,' she said. I gave her a squeeze and walked her out to reception, back to her daughter.

I watched as they went to their vehicle in the grey car park and then turned and made my way towards Ralph. I kneeled by his head and gave him a final scratch behind the ears. 'You were a much-loved dog, Ralph – your mum thought the world of you, little man,' I whispered into his ear. I spun on my heel and started to walk back to the prep room. I was just getting back to the hustle and bustle as I felt my eyes start to water. I dived into the nearest cupboard, the little cupboard under the stairs where the computer server was kept. I pulled the door behind me just as I started to bawl floods of tears. I slumped down the wall as I let the emotion wash over me; I had been keeping it in all day but now there was no stopping it. I cried for what felt like fifteen minutes, proper tears falling onto my scrub trousers, and all I kept replaying in my head was what I had overheard Mrs Johns' daughter promising her that morning in the car park. I had broken that promise.

I called my mum on the way home and told her about my day. She sat on the other end of the phone in silence, listening. When I finally stopped blubbing, she took a deep sigh. 'Oh darling, that must have been so hard.' She always says the right thing, my mum. We went on to have a proper catch-up and before I knew it I was pulling up back at my flat. I thanked my mum for being a sounding board (something she would do countless times over the next five years) and sharing my grief, and went upstairs. It had been a tough first day but I fell asleep thinking about the happy Boxer dog. I could almost hear the thud of his tail.

6

Survival Instincts

My career had started with a bang, I flew straight into emergency work and loved it. Yes, there were days like the one with Ralph, but mostly it was exciting, high energy, and I felt like I had really found my calling. Night shifts are something that split opinion in veterinary. As a student you are made to work night shifts on occasion to get a taste of what it's like in the real vet world. There are generally two kinds of students: those that loved it and thrived on the buzz and adrenaline (which was me) and those who walked around bleary eyed, not doing much, eventually finding a comfy dog bed to have a sleep on. I knew then, pretty early on in my rotations, that night work was something I wanted to experience in the real world. I think that for some students the prospect of night work, with emergencies being the majority of the cases you will see, can seem daunting. I certainly had friends in my final year who thought I was crazy, wanting to get stuck in to emergency work so early in my career. I started looking for positions where night work was a large part of the job description, whilst the majority of my classmates tried their hardest to find jobs with no night work at all, wanting to find their feet before getting emergency experience. There is no right approach to this and I'm sure I was a little mad to go for it so early on, but it was what I wanted to do.

The hospital where I took my first job (and the place I met Ralph the Boxer) was indeed open twenty-four hours, three hundred and sixty-five days a year. I very quickly found myself working nights and I loved it. There was something about the buzz, something about the emergency nature of the work. I would be sitting in my scrubs, stethoscope round my neck, one of the only people awake, ready to look out for and help the animals in their time of need. It was exhilarating. The calls to the vets would vary hugely. I started playing a bit of a game with the other night vets – who got the phone call from the furthest away. The clinic was called 'West Vets', a pretty generic name, and due to the wonderful tech team in the office we had a pretty good presence on search engines and social media. This meant that when people googled 'emergency vet' or 'night vet', our clinic was regularly the first hit. In blind panic at two o'clock in the morning, people would regularly just press 'Call' on their mobile phone and end up speaking to me or my colleagues. After a few instances of this, we started answering the phone, 'West Vets Emergency, may I ask where you're calling from?' But before we started this we ended up with some rather hilarious calls. One of my friends had a call from a very confused Scottish woman in Glasgow, clearly not understanding my colleague's

Spanish accent, as he tried to explain to her that her cat would likely die before she made it the 430 miles to Kent. The rest of the team regularly got calls from far up north – Liverpudlian, Mancunian and Birmingham accents all being regular findings on the other end of the emergency phone.

One night the phone rang at about 11pm. We had recently had a meeting about the long-distance calls we were getting more and more of, so I dutifully answered the phone, 'Good evening, West Vets Emergency, may I ask where you're calling from please?'

The confused woman on the end of the phone stumbled a bit, slightly taken aback at being asked where she was, and replied, 'Oh, um, Kent County.'

She had what I thought was an American accent, so I excused her use of 'Kent County' and carried on the call: 'Okay, how can I help?'

'Um, well, I am trying to find your entrance but I can't seem to see you guys,' she explained.

'Ah, okay, no worries, where abouts are you? What can you see? Are you anywhere near the Tesco?'

'Tesco?' She sounded perplexed. 'I don't know what that is, but don't worry, I think I've found you.'

'Okay, well, if you pull up and ring the bell I will meet you in the reception,' I said. It is commonplace to keep the building locked up and only answer to clients over the intercom – after all there are thousands of pounds worth of drugs in veterinary clinics.

This seemed to confuse the lady. 'Wait, can I not just walk in?' she asked.

'No, I'm afraid at this time of night we keep the building locked up. But don't worry, just ring the bell.'

Somehow this seemed to confuse her further. 'But I can see people in there – I don't understand what you mean,' she said.

'Where are you calling from? Our reception is closed and only the nursing staff and I are in the clinic,' I said.

'I told you, I'm calling from Kent County,' she said in mild frustration.

I started to twig. 'Kent County, where?' I asked.

'Kent County, Ontario, of course.' The American accent I had picked up was in fact a Canadian one.

'Right, I think you have called the wrong clinic. This is a vet's just outside London in England.' She apologised and I wished her well with her animal. I had a bit of a google once we were off the phone and indeed, there was a 'West Vets' in Kent County, Ontario, in Canada. Safe to say, I won the competition with my colleagues.

*

It wasn't all fun and games – working nights can really test you. Some nights would be quiet for the first few hours, to be followed by a flurry of calls within about half an hour of each other. Other nights you would be in back-to-back consults from the start of the shift at eight in the evening all the way through until one in the morning. Then again some nights were just plain mad.

I was about a year out of university, still finding my feet as a vet and really enjoying my emergency work. I had seen my fair share of emergencies on my night shifts: dogs hit by cars, cats having been missing for days finally turning up at two in the morning with fight wounds all over them, having to perform life-saving surgery on critically ill animals. You name it, I had done it, or at least I thought so. I got a call at about midnight – it was from a guy called Alex who sounded rather distressed but I couldn't decipher quite what was going on. I caught little snippets of what had happened and tried to piece it together: 'don't know what happened', 'Mum started shouting', 'accusing me of abuse', 'stormed out', 'dog been stabbed' . . .

At this point I interjected. 'Wait, wait, wait Alex, what was that last bit – you have a dog and it's been stabbed?' I asked forcefully, trying to stop the man on the other end from continuing to blab. It had the desired effect.

'Yes,' he replied simply.

'Okay, what was he stabbed with? Where has he been stabbed? How long ago did this happen? How does the dog seem?' I fired the questions down the phone at him, then realised I was probably going a few steps at once. 'Sorry, Alex, let's start again. How is the dog in himself?'

'He seems okay, mate, he's just sorta' lying there.'

'Okay, and what was he stabbed with – is it still in him?' I thought he could probably handle those two questions at once.

'A knife and no, it's out. He might have been stabbed a few times in the stomach.' He was getting good at this: three questions at once.

'Right, okay, and is there any bleeding?' I followed up.

'A bit but not much,' he replied.

'Okay, Alex, that's great, now listen closely – what I need you to do is wrap him tightly in a blanket, especially around his abdomen, and then bring him straight in to see me.'

He agreed and he told me he would be about twenty minutes. I could hear his mother arguing in the background, but as Alex hung up I was happy that he understood the plan and he was going to do his best to get here as soon as he could.

I spent the next ten minutes gathering all the emergency drugs and equipment that I would need with one of the night nurses. Blood tubes, syringes, needles, the ECG, oxygen mask, pain relief and everything to put the dog under general anaesthetic in case we needed to go straight into theatre. I was just about finished when the phone rang again. I answered it while drawing up some emergency drugs into a syringe and nearly dropped the bottle of adrenaline when the person on the other end started talking. 'Hi there, this is PC Baker from North Kent police. I believe you had a gentleman on the phone just now with a dog that's been stabbed – is that correct?'

I put the needle and syringe down and sat on the desk. 'Yes, that's right. I think his name was Alex. Is everything okay?' I asked. My voice had gone all shaky as if I had done something wrong.

'Okay, so we have just had a 999 call from his mother – apparently Alex has a history of mental illness and it was in fact him who stabbed the dog.' My face must have been a picture because Natalie, the nurse I was on overnight with, suddenly stopped what she was doing and stared at me.

'Okay,' I replied, not really knowing what to say or do in this sort of situation.

The police officer went on, 'We have ascertained that we don't think he is dangerous but we don't want you to inter-act with him.'

'No shit,' I thought. I wasn't exactly keen on chatting about the weather with a man who had just stabbed his own dog multiple times anyway. 'So what should I do?' I asked. The policeman went on to explain that there were units on the way now, hopefully in time to beat Alex to the clinic. He explained that he wanted me to stay inside the reception and watch until it was safe to open the door and come out to get the dog. If Alex beat the officers there, I was to take the dog from him and leave him outside of the vet's until offic-ers arrived to arrest him. I much preferred the idea of having the police there before he arrived. I confirmed the plan with the officer and went to the reception to wait. The reception was quite big, probably about 50ft long and glass-fronted. This meant I could sit just inside and see everything that was going on in the car park, even with the blinds pulled over.

About five minutes passed and I watched as a black Ford Focus pulled into the car park. There were no police lights anywhere to be seen and my stomach tightened at the thought of having to face the dog stabber alone. I walked slowly to the door as the car pulled up just outside, the darkness shrouding the figures in the car. Both front doors swung open and out got two men, in stab vests with body cams attached; the police had beaten Alex. I felt my stomach relax and went to open the reception door. I let the police officers in and introduced myself. They took me through what they thought was going to happen; they had two more officers on the way and another on standby just in case. Now the 'muscle' had arrived I suddenly felt much calmer about the whole situation. In fact, a small part of me was actually starting to enjoy the adrenaline rush that came along with the nerves.

We agreed that when Alex arrived, we would wait for him to get out of the car and then the police officers would approach him. Once they had ascertained that Alex was no threat, I would rush out and grab the dog, running back inside with him to start working on him to, hopefully, save his life. I had never dealt with a stab wound before and I felt a bit like a human doctor working on *24 hours in A&E*. Of course I had seen lacerations and big wounds before – they had been some of my favourite and most rewarding cases. They often posed quite a surgical dilemma, drawing on your skill as a vet to pick the best way to close the skin to give the animal the greatest chance of healing without complications. What those procedures had all had in common, however, was that not a single one of them had been intentional – they were almost exclusively accidents where the dog or cat had caught itself on something sharp or accidentally run into something whilst out on a walk. This one was inflicted with a sharp implement, by a human being. I suddenly felt sick as it started to really dawn on me what was going on. I was now in charge of saving the life of a dog that had been abused by its owner. Yes, its owner may have mental illness, but essentially this was a case of animal abuse. My thought process was cut short as a set of headlights entered the car park and swung round into a space. The officers stood up and went to the door. They waited for the figure driving the car to get out and suddenly they sprung into action.

Before I knew what was happening, the officers were charging down the car, with two more officers having appeared at the entrance to the carpark. I caught my first glimpse of Alex as he turned towards the shouting policemen, his pale face enhanced by the moonlight. He was about 5ft 10in, dressed head to toe in a grey Nike tracksuit, with sharp features and small dark eyes that looked as if he trusted no-one. He was glancing between the officers, his face one of panic. I watched from a safe distance as he tried to work out what was going on. I think I knew he was going to try to run before even he did, and, sure enough, a few seconds later he made straight for a gap between the police officers. The policemen converged on the man like the defensive line of a rugby team and in a matter of moments they had Alex on the floor with his arms behind his back.

One of the officers was cuffing him as I was broken from my trance by shouts of 'Hey you, vet guy!' from my left. I had completely forgotten there was a dog to be seen to and I kicked myself for taking my eye off the ball. I tore my gaze away from the commotion and ran over to the car. There was a large male Staffordshire bull terrier lying on the back seat of the car; he had a chain collar around his neck with a big garish tag that read 'King'. When I say 'large', he was massive, weighing in at easily 25kg. I tried to assess the situation – there was a little blood on the white blanket wrapped around the dog but he was conscious and holding his head up, clearly interested in what was happening out in the car park. I held a hand out and the dog sniffed me, his tail went and he gave me a gentle lick. I took this to mean that he wouldn't try to take my arm off and managed to scoop him up into my arms. I carried him through to the prep room with one of the policemen. The nurses were waiting and we got to work.

King had three stab wounds in a line, from just behind his rib cage back to the level of his belly button (or umbilicus if you're feeling fancy). I traced them with my finger like a morbid 'join the dots' – the wounds were all about a centimetre and had dried blood around them. I gave him some pain relief and had a gentle look at the wounds. From the outside you would have thought he was actually okay, but he was telling me a different story. After carrying him in, I had placed him on an examination table and he had slumped over onto his side. He was still lying in that position, his chest rising and falling faster than it should have been. I poked gently at the wounds. As far as I could tell with King conscious, the knife had gone all the way into his abdomen on the first stab, the wound that was the furthest forward, but not on the second two – they were only muscle deep. This was good news, but I was still worried about what damage that first stab had done.

I found myself wondering what the scene would have been like at home with him and Alex. Had the man attacked the dog, catching him unawares with the first stab, the dog being too quick to allow the second and third attempts to cause as much damage? I was playing it over in my head and had to snap myself out of it. I checked his mouth – his gums were pale, and Natalie the nurse took his temperature, telling me he was on the cold side. Natalie was a seasoned pro at emergency work. I felt like I knew what to do in most emergencies, but having such an experienced nurse with me always gave me that comfort blanket. She was incredible to watch, taking King's pulse and temperature while getting a blanket and setting up fluids: it was like she had seventeen pairs of hands. As more pieces of the puzzle came together, I became more and more sure that he was bleeding internally. I ran through to the imaging suite and wheeled the ultrasound machine through the prep room to the side of the dog. I popped the probe on his abdomen and was greeted by a black screen swirling around on the monitor. I was right: he had an abdomen full of blood. 'Shit,' I said out loud, looking at the black abyss on the screen.

The policeman heard and was immediately interested. 'What's up, fella?' he asked in a relaxed tone that I have only ever really heard from a copper.

'We are going to have to go in,' I said, turning to look at him. 'It doesn't look good.' Until that point, the policeman had just been taking photographs on his phone, presumably for evidence, not just because he was interested, and, after I told him what was next, he radioed in to his colleagues to give them an update. As he went off to do so, I turned to start putting the dog under anaesthetic. He was fading fast and the quicker we could get into theatre, the better chance we had of saving him. Natalie started prepping the surgical field, and I moved over to the scrub sink to sterilise my hands and suddenly had a dilemma. 'Who was going to fund this?' I thought to myself. It's a wonderful thing, the NHS, but it doesn't half put vets in a sticky situation sometimes.

A remarkable number of people think there is some sort of animal NHS – meaning they don't have to pay for treatment. As much as I would love it, I can assure you there isn't. Don't be mistaken, there is rarely a proper answer to who's funding these cases. Most clinics will have a policy on these sorts of things but not even we, a well-organised emergency clinic, had a policy on treating animals where the owner had been arrested. It would be a lovely reality to be able to perform life-saving treatment and surgery for my patients without anyone having to foot the bill but, alas, that is not the case. I suddenly felt uneasy – usually this was a conversation I would have with an owner, but Alex was rather preoccupied at the moment being wrestled into the back of a police car. I had two options: one, face my boss with an insane story in the morning and slyly drop in that I hadn't actually taken any money from anyone; or two, ask the slightly scary policeman who was going to pay for the surgery when he came back from talking to his colleagues. The policeman came back as I was finishing scrubbing up and I, of course, wussed out, and took option one. Money was tomorrow's problem.

We were in theatre within fifteen minutes. The dog was incredibly stable for an animal with most of its circulating blood volume within its abdomen. I threw a drape over his tummy, now starting to bulge with the sheer pressure building from the fluid. 'Okay, here we go; make sure you have that suction ready,' I said, directing the second part of my sentence at the kennel hand who I had made scrub in to help me. Kennel assistants are exactly what it says on the tin – they are helpers in the kennels. What they are not is a spare pair of hands in a surgical procedure, but hey, I needed someone and it was either her or the policeman. I made my first cut and popped through the layers into the peritoneum. Bright red blood spilled out as soon as I did so and started to flow down both sides of the dog's abdomen. I grabbed the suction from my assistant and plunged the instrument into the depths of the dog's belly. Suction is an odd concept – you will have seen it on TV if you watch medical shows. It is essentially a glorified medical hoover, used to remove blood from your surgical field so you can see what you're doing. In this case, the machine was working overtime, removing a steady flow of blood, and as it did so I started to look around the abdomen to try to find the origin of the huge amount of blood. There aren't many places in the abdomen that could cause such a large bleed so quickly, so I started making a list in my head. I found the entrance of the knife from the inside of the dog and tried to visualise where it would have passed through. I was beginning to mock myself for wasting time with silly visualisation when my eye caught what looked like a spray of blood. I moved my suction tip over to the area, pulled the spleen back (what an odd sentence) and had a closer look. I stood there, slightly taken aback as I saw the extent of the damage.

The knife had passed through King, wreaking havoc. The blood was spilling out from a slice through his spleen but, unfortunately, that was the least of his worries. On its way to his spleen, the knife had passed through King's stomach, his pancreas and almost bisected one of his kidneys. I looked at Natalie and she immediately knew: this was borderline unfixable.

Ask anyone who works with animals and they will tell you: sometimes animals just know. They know how you're feeling, they know what you're doing and they absolutely know what you're thinking. King knew. Even from the depths of his anaesthetic, King knew. He knew he wasn't going to make it but he had hung on just long enough to show me what had happened. The reason I say this is because as I looked up to Natalie with a look of 'Holy shit', he let go. His body, which had been through so much, gave up. His ECG flat-lined and we started CPR to try to get him back. In these sorts of cases, however, I sometimes find myself thinking, do we really want to get him back? Don't get me wrong, he seemed like a lovely dog, but would it be fair to him to bring him back? His owner, the person he trusted most in the world, had betrayed him in the ultimate way. He had been through incredible amounts of pain, with multiple organ damage. He was likely going to need a splenectomy (removal of the spleen), an enterectomy (removal of parts of the intestine), a partial or full nephrectomy (removal of part of, or a whole kidney), and that was just for starters. He would have weeks of recovery, and it was impossible to know if he would survive. Then, and this is the bit I wasn't entirely sure about, he would likely have to spend time in police kennels, where he would be used as evidence in the prosecution of his owner. The poor dog in front of me had been through a lot, and he would have so much more pain and suffering if he survived.

I took my surgical hat, mask and gloves off. I slumped down in the corner of the room and put my head in my hands. I sat there and tried to wipe my mind clean of the horror that I had just seen. I was suddenly angry, seething at what the poor dog had been put through. How had this man been allowed to own a dog? Why did the country not have tighter laws on dog ownership? I stormed out of theatre, ripping my surgical gown off as I went and found a quiet place where I could sit and try to calm down.

Later, I gave a statement to the police and they said they would be in touch the next day. I didn't ask but I was sure that this could end up with me in court giving my witness account. I was still angry about what had happened, but it was coming up for two o'clock in the morning by this point and, despite the adrenaline rush of the last few hours, my body and mind were tired. I said goodbye to the policemen and stood in the car park as they left. I looked up at the night sky – it was overcast but not so much that you couldn't see the stars. I stood there for a few minutes and let the calm wash over me, before heading back inside to help clear up from the mayhem.

I often wonder what ever happened to Alex. I was called by the police to clarify a few things and add in extra comments to my statement over the next few weeks, but the trail went cold after that. I never heard of a court date or anything more about the man that had stabbed his dog to death. I have seen some pretty horrific surgical cases over the years: dogs and cats with tumours invading almost every organ in the body, winding their way around blood vessels, gripping the body like an angel of death. I've seen dogs with open wounds almost the size of their entire body, and cats with tumours growing out of their eyes. Nothing has come close, though, to the horror I felt that night. It wasn't the damage to the dog that was harrowing – it was the fact that it was the owner who did it.

*

Animals in pain are tough to think about. My girlfriend is the worst at it. I regularly come home and talk about my day at work, wanting to share in the weird and wonderful things I've seen, but she can't think about it and runs away before I show her a 'gross photo'. She can't handle the idea of animals hurting, let alone not being able to communicate such things. But what I really struggle with, as I'm sure most of us do, is animal cruelty.

I'm not sure how I classify what happened that night. Alex was clearly unwell, with mental illness, so is it his fault that he killed his pet? If it isn't his fault, then whose is it? Is it his parent's fault for allowing him to own a dog? Is it the government's fault for not having tighter dog ownership laws? Should we bring back the dog licence? I don't think there is a right answer to this but it is something that we need to think about.

Animal cruelty sentencing is a bit of a joke. Until recently, the maximum sentence for acts of animal cruelty in the UK was six months. Six measly months for abusing, threatening and undoubtedly killing animals. I am honoured to have been appointed as an RSPCA ambassador, and they are working tirelessly to help improve the welfare of animals in the UK. I cannot imagine the horrors some RSPCA inspectors have to deal with on a daily basis, and I count myself very lucky to work in a part of the country where I see very little animal cruelty.

Treacle, the most gorgeous lemon cocker spaniel puppy, came into my life a few years ago and unfortunately served as a reminder that there are bad people out there.

*

Treacle had been picked up by my clients a day before coming in to see me. We regularly see puppies in the few days following their new owners collecting them. We check them over and make sure everything is okay before they get settled into their new home. Many good breeders out there get the puppies checked over before they are picked up, but it is a good idea to get your own vet's opinion just in case. So that's exactly what was planned for that morning: Treacle was coming in to see me with her owners, Tracy and Mel, who were keen to show off their pride and joy. They had an appointment booked for ten o'clock, so I was a bit surprised when they rocked up at half past eight, just as I was finishing my first consult of the morning. The look of concern on their faces was enough to stop me in my tracks, so I guided them straight into my consult room to see what was wrong.

'She's really listless, Rory,' said Tracy, as she unfurled the bundle of blankets from her chest onto the table. Inside the blankets was a puppy, curled up in a ball, shivering with every breath.

'She's not right,' I said. 'What's happened?' They explained that they had been to pick up the puppy the day before and she had been okay but slept most of the evening. She hadn't eaten her dinner and then, this morning, she was just like this – curled up, shivering. 'How old is she meant to be?' I asked the mums.

'Nine weeks,' they replied in unison. There was no way this pup was nine weeks, I thought to myself as I gently popped her onto the scales in the consult room. The screen on the scales flashed up 2.1kg: she was less than half the weight I would expect for a nine-week-old.

'Did you see the other puppies?' I asked. The two women looked at each other.

'No,' Mel said sheepishly, knowing that I wasn't going to like the answer. 'We did think it was a bit weird, but we weren't allowed to go and see the puppies before we picked her up and when we went yesterday they brought her to us.'

'Okay, so you didn't see the mum?' They shook their heads. 'And do you have any record of a vaccination or vet check?' I asked hopefully.

Their faces lit up. 'Oh yes, we have a vaccine card. Here.' Mel produced a folded piece of card with a picture of a dog on the front. I opened the card and inspected it. There were two vaccine bottle stickers in the middle of the page with a scribble that I assumed was a signature next to them.

There was no microchip number in the card and the name was written in as 'Puppy 1'. There was no vet stamp. I dismissed the vaccine card, taking it from the owners to inspect properly later on, and got back to the matter at hand.

'Okay, you're going to have to leave Treacle with me. I don't know exactly what is wrong with her but she is definitely not right.' The women were very upset. What was meant to be a happy week filled with puppy cuddles and cuteness had taken a real turn and was now becoming a bit of a week from hell. They cooed over Treacle as we said goodbye and I rushed the little puppy into the prep room.

*

Puppies, as you'll know, are usually bright and bouncy little things. They are bundles of energy, biting fingers and noses and licking your ears to death. This one was most definitely not that. She was curled up, shaking, hardly paying attention to anyone or anything – she was not well. I placed an IV in her leg and took some blood. If there is one thing to test in a listless pup, it's their glucose (sugar levels) and, as the monitor beeped into action, I was not surprised when it told me that Treacle's level was dangerously low. I gave her a bolus (a single dose injection) of glucose and started her on some fluids. With puppies it can be tricky not to overload them: you have to be very careful with rates of fluids and medications as the slightest mistake can push their fragile little bodies too far, causing more harm than good. I sat with the little puppy on my knee, wrapped in a blanket and waited for the rest of her blood tests to come through. When I had brought Treacle through to the prep room, I had donned my fashionable plastic apron and gloves. I had also made the nurse helping me do the same. I had not explained why because I didn't want to entertain the thought, though the rest of the team knew exactly what I was worried about.

Parvovirus is probably one of the worst infectious diseases we see in the UK. You see it in the press every so often when an outbreak wipes out a few litters of puppies. 'PUPPY KILLER VIRUS' splashed across the pages of the newspapers sparking mass panic amongst vets and dog owners alike. I had only seen cases a few times, never had one of my own, and every single fibre of my being wanted it to stay that way. Parvo is a horrible disease that causes puppies to, for want of a better phrase, shit their guts out. It is so severe that often you can see bits of gut lining coming out with each squirt of liquid diarrhoea. This process has a rather particular smell, leading to vets across the country often suggesting that one can smell a case of parvo before you see it. I waited impatiently as the parvovirus snap test (a type of diagnostic test used to give a quick diagnosis from a few drops of blood) sat on the side, the blood slowly creeping across the test field. I had to wait fifteen minutes for the answer and busied myself writing my clinical notes, with Treacle still curled up in a ball on my lap. As the minute hand finally crept round on the clock, I walked over to where the test was and glanced at the lines in front of me. Snap tests are a bit like pregnancy tests: they have a control line and a test positive line. In this test two lines was bad, one line was good. One line greeted me and I let out a sigh of relief that I wasn't even aware I was holding in; Treacle didn't have parvo.

The rest of her blood results came through later and we spent the day intensively monitoring her for improvement. She had spent the majority of the morning sleeping but after a few hours she perked up. She even showed interest in some food when I went to offer it to her. I sat with her as she gently licked the food off of my fingers, one little nibble at a time. She was so small – definitely not nine weeks of age: my guess was closer to five. As the day went on she got stronger and stronger and I fell more and more in love with the little puppy. I had her in my lap later that day while I was doing more paperwork and I should really have been wearing an apron because, although she didn't have parvovirus, she could still have had something else that was infectious.

One of the senior nurses had just told me off for putting her in my lap (nurses really do run the show in a vet's) and, as I turned to retort, I heard a squelch from below. I froze and looked down as she produced a jet of liquid diarrhoea all over my crotch. The problem with being sat down is that you immediately want to get up and remove the offending animal from your lap. However, as this puppy was so unwell, I needed a sample of her stool to send for diagnostics. So I sat there and let it happen. Once the puppy was done, the same nurse who had told me off sauntered over with a beaming smile on her face and whisked the puppy back to her kennel. I was given a sample pot and had to sort of shimmy to manoeuvre some of the foetid brown sludge from my lap into the container. I mopped the rest of the diarrhoea from my lap and headed upstairs for a shower. Thank God we have a shower at work.

Not even this managed to put me off the little bundle of fluff. By the time I sent her back home to her mums later that evening she was a much happier puppy. She had eaten a small amount of food and her glucose levels had come up to a much better level.

The next day, I started my detective work. This puppy was most definitely not as old as the breeder had said and there was something not right about the way that Mel and Tracy had been sold their puppy. I started with the vaccine card. It was tattered and looked old, not a brand new one like you would usually expect with a puppy. I turned the piece of card over in my hands trying to find a clue about which vet had given the document out. On the back, there was a small square of branding which gave the veterinary surgery name and a phone number which I punched into the phone keypad. I spoke to a lovely, cheery receptionist who had the kind of voice that puts a smile on your face. I told her the story and gave her the breeder's name and she looked up the file. Due to GDPR (General Data Protection Regulation) she couldn't give me a huge amount of information, but what she did let slip was that the person hadn't been into the vet's with puppies and she most definitely hadn't been seen in the last six months. Why then, I wondered, did I have a vaccine card dated last week with vaccine stickers on it, supposedly belonging to Treacle? I thanked her and hung up. I often wonder what other vets do in these situations. Do they just let it lie or are they like me, a dog with a bone who just can't let it go?

The story that Mel and Tracy had told me had all the hallmarks of a dodgy breeder, and now that the puppy was ill and the vaccine card seemed like it could be a fake, I was really concerned we were dealing with a puppy farm. Puppy farms are like hell on earth. I must admit that I am glad to have never set foot in one, but I have seen enough photos and heard enough horror stories to tell you that I absolutely never want to witness one first-hand. Dogs kept in cages, hardly able to move in the tiny confines of their prisons. Mothers forced to have litter after litter of puppies, often to the point of exhaustion and ultimately death. The puppies raised in crappy conditions, covered in urine and faeces and eventually shipped off to a new home, regularly taken from their mothers far too early. One of the worst things I have ever heard was from an RSPCA inspector friend of mine. He was out raiding a puppy farm with the police, and in one of these utter hell-holes he found a cat carrier. On first look, this particular cat carrier seemed to be chock full of something furry and it was very heavy. He removed the top of the carrier and revealed something truly harrowing: a Newfoundland puppy.

Newfoundland puppies are rather large things, much bigger than your average cat. The monsters that had been running this puppy farm had popped the puppy into the carrier and promptly forgotten about him. He had grown to the point where he was so tightly confined that he could no longer breathe and when my friend eventually found him, he was very, very dead. The suffering that these places use to make a profit is almost unrivalled in its cruelty, so I had a sick feeling in the pit of my stomach when I started to wonder if Treacle had started her life in one such place.

*

I reported the breeder to the RSPCA. I wanted to drive around to her house and break in to have a snoop, but that would have been highly illegal. I have reported a few incidents to the RSPCA in my time, the first of which was when I was just ten years old. I had taken it upon myself to call the RSPCA as I felt the sheep in the field next to us weren't being looked after terribly well. I regularly looked out and saw sheep lying on their sides with their feet in the air. I was hugely concerned about their welfare and saw no other option than to get in touch with the RSPCA. I wasn't sure how seriously the lady on the end of the phone had taken me with my squeaky pre-pubescent voice, but I hung up the phone feeling like I had done some good. A week later, I spotted the farmer in the field and went out to talk to him. I explained what had happened and what I had seen. To my surprise, he had burst into laughter, clearly amused by the fact that it was a ten-year-old that had got in touch with the RSPCA. He walked me over to one of the sheep on its side and told me to roll her onto her belly. I did as I was told, heaving the pregnant ewe onto its front. It sat there and steadied itself before letting out an almighty burp, getting up and wandering off to find some tasty grass. The farmer told me that it was something that occasionally happened and, from that day forward, I was chief sheep tipper if I was to ever see a sheep on its side. As sweetly as that turned out, I don't enjoy reporting people to the RSPCA: I feel almost like I'm telling tales, but sometimes it's the last thing a vet can do to protect animal welfare.

Often, these reports go no further, like the time I reported a seventy-year-old woman, and no, I didn't feel bad about it. She had come in to see me with her new kitten. Like most kittens, he was full of beans, causing mischief and getting into trouble. Over the weekend he had decided that he wanted to see out of the window, a particularly high window with a radiator underneath it. After working out how to scale the curtain he had tried to flip himself onto the window ledge but, unfortunately, he had misjudged the landing (as kittens often do) and fallen and caught his leg behind the radiator. Now, ordinarily cats are pretty good at landing on their feet, but this little chap managed to fall at such an angle that he snapped his radius and ulna clean in half. The owner had luckily seen this happen and recovered the cat from behind the radiator. I would like to think that most of you reading this book would, if that unfortunate situation were to happen to you and your pet, go straight to the vet's. This lovely old dear decided that in fact, it was better not to do so and to wait until Monday morning, over twenty-four hours later. I struggled to hide my shock as she told me this, my face making some warped grimace. I picked up the kitten and pointed out the break to the owner. I often give the benefit of the doubt to people for missing things with their pets but this was impossible to miss: the poor little chap's paw was just flapping in the breeze. At this point I told the owner that we would really need to X-ray to see the extent of the damage and the cat needed pain relief, lots and lots of pain relief. The owner simply looked at me and said, 'Oh no dear, that won't be necessary, God told me that if I just give him time, it will heal.'

Cue a thirty-minute argument back and forth between me and the owner discussing the need for the cat to have some pain relief. She became indignant with me, refusing to give me permission to administer the pain relief and saying that I was going against God's will and suggesting unnecessary things. You may at this point think that this was because the owner could not afford treatment but no, she had an all-singing, all-dancing insurance policy for the cat. God had a lot to answer for. So yes, I reported her to the RSPCA. Unfortunately, I didn't ever hear what happened to that poor, poor cat and crazy God lady.

*

Treacle was getting better. She had a cocktail of medications that seemed to be helping and a few days later I had her faecal results back. She had a Yersinia infection, something I had never seen before. Yersinia is a genus of bacteria that causes disease in a number of animals. The strain of Yersinia that Treacle had was 'enterocolitica', which causes vomiting and diarrhoea. A form of Yersinia you may be more familiar with is *Yersinia pestits*, more commonly known as the bacteria that caused the plague. As well as this, Treacle had a salmonella infection, campylobacter and coccidiosis. I sat at the computer reading through the results, my mouth open, hardly able to believe the amount of positive results that had come through. She had pretty much every infectious gastrointestinal disease going (except parvo thank goodness). She had to be a puppy farm dog; only a puppy from that sort of background could live in conditions harbouring so many diseases. I called Treacle's owners and let them know the score. They were completely on board with the report to the RSPCA, and I called the inspector on the case and gave him the faecal results. Every part of me hoped that there would be a reason for this, one that didn't involve suffering dogs, but my gut was telling me that this was the start of something bigger than Treacle. Days dragged on into weeks and eventually, upon hearing nothing more, I conceded that the trail had gone cold.

Mel and Tracy were none the wiser either. Six months passed and I was all but ready to write it off. There is only so much you can do: I had treated Treacle and she was now a bouncy adolescent. Without knowing her history, you would never have known she'd been such a poorly pup. Then, one morning as I sat on the counter behind reception chatting to the receptionists, Mel came bursting through the clinic door. 'You won't believe it, Rory –' she started, 'they only went and raided the place!'

It took me a minute to work out what she was on about – I hadn't even had my first coffee of the day – but as I put two and two together I jumped off the counter. 'What?! That's amazing news!' I half shouted back, almost throwing my coffee over Mel in my excitement.

'Yeah, it's brilliant. But the awful thing is, apparently there were all sorts of dogs there: they seized almost fifty animals!'

'Treacle saved them – she told us there was a problem and she has saved those other animals,' I said, getting slightly carried away. But, in a way, Treacle had.

She had escaped the horrible place and brought with her a trail of clues leading back to a disgusting puppy farm that now, thanks to her and a bunch of other puppies, was a thing of the past. Treacle still comes to see me to this day and she is the most wonderful, gentle dog. When I think of the horrors she went through at such a young age, at the hand of a human being, and to now be so trusting and gentle . . . dogs really are special.

7

Three Legs Are Better Than Four

I had read and re-read the textbook ten times. I could see the diagram of the Y-shaped incision encircling the hind leg, but still I stood there, scalpel to skin, not moving . . . All of my training had faded to a distant whisper in the back of my mind. I had performed this surgery a mere two weeks before with no issue, and here I was stood with a gormless look on my face, as if I shouldn't be allowed to pet an animal, let alone take a scalpel to one.

'I haven't felt this much pressure in surgery forever!' I mumbled to my nurse through my surgical mask as my mouth started to dry up like the Gobi desert. We were the only two people in the room, yet I felt like I was being watched, probably not helped by the glass-walled surgical theatre making the room look like a new feature at the London aquarium. I shuffled uncomfortably as I started to bake under the million-watt surgical light. I closed my eyes. 'Deep breath, Rory –' I encouraged myself, 'sort yourself out.' I thought back to the hundreds, possibly thousands, of times I had put scalpel to skin – how was this any different? I will tell you why it was different: because for the first time,

I was madly in love with the creature lying in front of me under anaesthetic.

We had got the call ten days before. 'There's a little cat in my porch and I think he is injured,' the lady at the end of the phone had explained to the receptionist. This isn't uncommon – we are in South London after all. When cats get hurt they generally have a very predictable reaction of run and hide. I wasn't in the clinic that day: I was on holiday sunning myself in the South of France, drinking Provencal rosé on the beach. The story was relayed to me in full as soon as I returned to work on a slightly glum Monday (you know, the first one back after a holiday).

The cat had been hit by a car, not far from the clinic where I was spending most of my consulting hours. He'd taken refuge in the kind woman's porch, and she had sensibly called and reported this to us.

'Can you pop him into the clinic?' my receptionist had asked.

There had been a pause on the other end of the phone. 'Umm . . . I think he might bite me,' had come the response. You may roll your eyes but, honestly, you can't blame her: injured cats are unpredictable and, if you aren't careful, a cat bite can put you in hospital.

'Okay, not a problem. Give us some time and we can organise someone to come and pick him up.'

An hour later and an amazing nurse had fetched the little fella and brought him into the clinic. On first assessment he was not having it, clearly very sore somewhere and not happy. Nothing some of the good drugs couldn't fix! After half an hour he was looking for a fuss and rolling around like a massive flirt. Cats are incredible: they often hide their pain, so much so that I colloquially refer to them as 'the great pretenders'.

One of my colleagues had quickly ascertained that he had a broken femur (thigh bone) and tibia (shin bone), and had bandaged him up with a 'Robert-Jones' (a type of bandage that immobilised the limb allowing for support and improved comfort while waiting for surgery or other treatment), the namesake of a trailblazing human orthopaedic surgeon from the turn of the 20th century.

I came back to work, ready to hit the ground running. Don't get me wrong, everyone needs a holiday once in a while (something I learnt the hard way after working for a year straight and almost pulling my hair out), but when you spend your days working with animals, you can only stay away so long. I count myself very lucky to love my job and I thank my dad for giving me some of the best advice I could have asked for as a kid. He always said to me as I was growing up, 'If you do something you love, you won't work a day of your life,' and oh how right he was.

I went straight to the cat ward and that's when I first met the little guy. He was curled up, sleeping, with his massive bandage sticking up in the air like a ship's sail. He was all black as far as I could see, very slight in build and he had a sheen to his coat that made it look almost fluid.

I popped a hand into the kennel to give him a bit of a fuss, and was greeted with a soft and hypnotic purr as he rolled onto his back and exposed a small patch of white on his chest. I took a look at his X-rays. 'Jesus,' I muttered, flicking backwards and forwards between the screens, 'for a cat with a leg *that* broken, he sure is friendly.' I kept fussing the little black cat. He was really, really lovely.

I went and grabbed a pouch of food from reception – I knew how to buy an animal's love. As I opened the kennel door and ripped open the pouch, he got up on all fours and almost tried to climb into my arms. I carried him back into the kennel, telling him to wait until I had at least got the pouch open. He sat there and looked up at me and I looked back at him. His eyes were quite possibly the biggest I had ever seen: deep, dark black surrounded by an incredible yellow ring. I'm not sure I had ever or have ever seen eyes quite like that before or since.

I slowly blinked at him* and he half-closed his eyes back at me and I was smitten. I put the whole pouch of food in a bowl and slid it into the kennel, and he was chowing down before the bowl had come to rest. I stayed and watched him for a bit, stroking him while he took big

---

* The 'much cleverer than I' cat specialists and behaviourists have recognised a behaviour in cats called the 'slow blink', which shows affection and comfort towards another cat or human. Whether or not a human can communicate it back to a cat is still up for debate, but for the sake of looking a bit weird in front of a client, I always slow blink at cats in the clinic.

mouthfuls of chicken. He was a bit like me – loved his food, and only really stopped between mouthfuls to give my hand a bit of a head rub.

I spent the whole day going backwards and forwards to the cat ward in-between consultations. I even got distracted fussing him while making up medications for a client, which my nurse ended up finishing for me with a wry smile (all hail super-nurses). Safe to say, the little guy kinda hindered my productivity.

Four more days passed, and I had started coming into work half an hour early just to make some time to play and fuss the little black cat. By this point he had spent nine days with us in the clinic with medications and bandages. My phone was full to the brim of photos of the little guy and my sister was getting seriously sick of hearing about him. I lived with Bethan at the time, the more impressive Cowlam sibling I may add. We had always been civil to each other as kids, not really loving or hating each other.

Of course we had our moments – like the time she pushed me down a flight of stairs leading to my first experience of local anaesthetic and stitches to sew together a gash in my head. Once we were in our early twenties though, we became best friends. Bethan is the smart one of the family – the sharpest of tongues and quickest wit making her a nightmare for her big brother to argue with, both qualities now being used to great effect as a London lawyer. She loves animals, but as I say, she was getting really sick of hearing about the stray cat at work.

When an animal comes into any vet surgery, routinely a member of staff will scan them for a microchip. Since April 2016 it has been a legal requirement for dogs over the age of eight weeks to be microchipped, yet somehow there is still no law for cats.

This little guy was unfortunately one of those who had slipped through the net. No microchip, but clearly with his temperament and condition he had an owner out there. We spent the whole time while he was with us popping photos of him on Facebook, Instagram, Twitter and anywhere else we could think of. We had clients reposting photos of him all over the internet, but sadly no-one came forward.

Microchips are wonderful things. They allow pets to be reunited with their owners every single day. In 2009, a study of over 7,700 animals showed that if you microchip your dog, you're more than twice as likely to be reunited if they wander off. But even more impressively than that, if you microchip your cat, you are twenty times more likely to see that little fluff ball again! The veterinary world is littered with amazing stories of how cats and dogs are reunited with owners after going missing.

Recently in our clinic we had a cat reunited with its owner. He had disappeared a few months previously from the owner's home in Cambridge. He had somehow turned up in Dulwich in South London. We had scanned his chip, contacted the owner and got him back home. Turns out he had taken a fancy to the matting in the back of a builder's van who had been doing some work on the house next door and taken a nap, only to wake up 70 miles away!

*

I remember in my second or third year of being a vet, I had a client bring in a cat. They had explained to me that she had 'just turned up' at their door a few years previously and 'sort of never left'. The cat had been named Tiggy, and quickly became a fully-fledged member of the family, coming and going as she pleased and demanding food on a regular basis. This happens more than you would think: cats can be fickle animals and they will regularly leave home like a surly teen-ager looking for a more suitable place to hang their hat. I have heard of cats leaving home for a huge number of reasons, usually including a new arrival such as a dog or a baby. One time I even had a client crying to me explaining that her beloved Reginald (yes, that's the cat) had packed up and left home because she had found herself a new man (a human boyfriend this time) and they 'just don't get on'.

Every vet out there will tell you that, at the very least, we hear of the local 'feeders' in the area. There is always some-one who insists on putting out food for the local 'strays', who actually aren't stray cats, just local residents on the prowl for more food. Tiggy, the new owner explained to me, had turned up one winter and started asking for food. The 'new' owner had kindly obliged with a tin of tuna and the rest was history. Two years down the line, and the owner had decided to bring her into the vet's for a health check and to see if she had a microchip. This also happens more than you might think. People become attached to animals (usually cats that visit their home), they give them cute names and then, before you know it, they're hoping they don't have owners so they can adopt them. By about two to three years into this sort of relationship, it often all becomes too much, and they need to know so they take them to the vet's.

Can I suggest, if you have a cat visiting you, either get them scanned by a vet (oh I don't know, possibly within a few weeks) or ask around the neighbours and try to find the rightful owner?

In this instance, the cat was in fine condition and, on examination, I couldn't find anything of concern with Tiggy. We did the whole vaccination chat and discussed the ins and outs of cat ownership. I wormed and flea-treated her and then I reached for the microchip scanner. 'Beep.' The scanner let out its familiar sound. The owner's face fell.

'Oh, does that mean she has another owner?' she asked.

'Well, it could do. You never know with these things; the chip might not be registered . . .' I suggested, trying not to break her heart. I put the fifteen-digit number into the database and, sure enough, up popped her given name (which most definitely wasn't Tiggy) and her rightful owner's telephone numbers and address. It turned out that the house Tiggy was registered to could be seen from the kitchen window of her new chosen home.

'So, do you have to call them?' the new owner asked.

'Um . . . well . . . yes, I do,' I replied, trying my utmost not to highlight the fact that she was asking me to essentially be a party to theft. The law regards all pets as property, so as much as I think the terms 'dog-napping' and 'cat-napping' should apply here, unfortunately, it's still just boring old theft.

I made an excuse about my consultation room phone not working, and left to go and call the old owner in private. I thumbed the number into the keypad and waited, hoping for the phone to have been disconnected or the number given incorrectly. This may seem wrong, but this cat had been living with my new client for the last two years, being looked after really well. If I could avoid the awkward 'your cat has been cheating on you' conversation, then that would be a win in my book.

Low and behold, the line started ringing and an abrupt woman answered the other end of the phone.

'Hi, my name is Rory and I'm a vet in South London,' I started.

'Yes?' she bit back, clearly questioning if I was really a vet or if this was the most elaborate PPI cover story ever.

'Well, I have just had one of my clients bring me your cat . . .'

'No, that's not possible, I have an indoor cat and I live in Norwich,' she said dismissively.

'Right, well the microchip I have just scanned gave me your name and number, and Tiggy, oh sorry, no . . .' I glanced at my computer screen, 'Mystique, is currently sitting on my consultation table,' I told her hurriedly, trying in the back of my mind to work out if she was a secret fan of X-men, or if she had just misspelt Mis-Teeq.

The line had gone quiet for a few seconds, 'What!' she came back to me, 'She can't be, she died . . .'

Well, there's a twist I didn't see coming. As it transpired, a few years back, Mystique had decided she'd had enough of being an indoor cat and one day, when her doting mother had left for work, she made a bid for freedom through the kitchen window. On returning to her now empty flat, her owner had gone full tilt making lost cat posters, posting over all social media channels known to man, calling all vets within a 10-mile radius, all unfortunately to no avail. Nobody had seen poor little Mystique, who was undoubtedly lost in the wilderness of South East London, starving hungry having not had her 4pm Dreamies.

Two long weeks passed and there was still no word, until one gloomy Monday morning the phone rang. The vet on the end of the line explained that they'd had a cat brought in over the weekend that matched Mystique's description. Unfortunately, the cat in question had decided to pick a fight with an articulated lorry and had lost in dramatic fashion, so much so that it was not entirely possible to tell if the cat had been male or female, let alone be sure if it was Mystique. With nothing else to go on, the owner had accepted her darling pet's fate, resigned herself to the fact that she would never see her again and had moved out of London.

Now, two years later, I was calling her and explaining that in fact, her cat was alive and well. She burst into tears. 'I thought she was deaaaaad,' came a wail down the phone.

Now I deal with my fair share of emotion in this job, but consoling a complete stranger from 100 miles away is a touch tricky. I gave her a minute to breathe and explained calmly that her cat had been living with a lovely lady who used to be her neighbour, was in perfect health and really a very sweet little thing. After a few minutes, she had composed herself and the inevitable question came next: 'So what do we do now?' she asked.

I have always struggled with the 'right thing to do' in these instances. Clearly, the cat still technically belongs to Miss Norwich, and it can all get a little nasty if not handled carefully. From experience, I find the best way is to leave it to the 'owners' to come to a conclusion and only get involved if entirely necessary. I popped Miss Norwich on hold and transferred her to my consult room.

Upon entering the room, the hopeful look on my client's face was soon wiped off when I explained the situation. I connected the call, handed the phone to her and left the room to let them chat. I busied myself looking down the microscope at a blood smear from one of my ongoing cases and got lost in the beauty of the white blood cells (honestly, they can be absolutely mesmerising).

When I returned to the consult room, I put Miss Norwich on speakerphone. 'So what have we decided?' I asked.

I am pleased to report that Tiggy still lives in South London with her new owner. It was very sensibly agreed that taking her up to Norwich and reverting her to an indoor cat, in a house that already had another cat, was likely to cause more harm than good. Better than that though, Miss Norwich got the train down to London and came and visited Tiggy (Mystique?) and her new owner, and even dropped into the clinic to say hello and give me a big box of chocolates. See? Microchips are always good.

The little injured black cat, who had found his way to our doorstep, was not as lucky as Tiggy. No microchip meant that the only option we had was to give him time for social media to work its magic and keep checking in with local vets to see if anyone had reported a missing feline. Despite his devilishly handsome face, no owner came forward, and on day ten of him being with us, we were resigned to the fact that we would have to discuss what to do with him.

I sat down with my bosses and we went through the options. I worked for (and still do) two Australian vets. They had both studied in 'Oz' and after separate time away from clinical practice, found themselves settling down in London at the same time. They had both experienced being overworked and the tough expectations of the veterinary world, so had started The Neighbourhood Vet with a view to it being more relaxed and a nice place to work. I love my bosses, and count myself very lucky to have a good working relationship with them and a friendship. I'm sure if they could, they would allow me to fix all the broken stray animals that came through our door, but at the end of the day we run a business and, as they told me that day, 'That is a surefire way to go bankrupt very quickly.' It is these sorts of cases that I have always found particularly tough. Working at independent clinics makes it a lot easier as, generally, I manage to twist my bosses' arms into allowing me to treat the animal for free, whether we find it a new home or not.

If we remove all emotion from these situations, generally there are three options. Firstly, we could euthanise the animal. It may sound harsh, it may sound cruel, but inherently, if there is no-one to look after the animal and it cannot look after itself, then euthanasia is a valid option (particularly, may I add, for those strays that aren't healthy). The next option is to find a place for the animal at a rescue centre. We are unbelievably privileged in this country to have a plethora of rescues willing to take on healthy and injured animals, and often treat them and then rehome them. To name a few, the RSPCA, Blue Cross and Battersea all do incredible work, and I truly believe the animals of the United Kingdom are lucky to have these amazing charities. Thirdly, and this would be the choice of most vets, although maybe not those who are business owners, is to treat the animal for free and then find the animal a new home.

If I owned my own clinic, I'm pretty sure I would be out of business after the first week. I am too soft, both on those who own their pets and also the strays and the wildlife that come in the door. I would treat and rehome every animal for free if I could; more than that, if I could I would treat all the animals out there for free. Charging for veterinary is not something that comes naturally to us animal-loving vets, and honestly that's half the issue with money and vets.

Anyway, that is beside the point here and, as we discussed the wee black cat, it became clear that we needed to treat his mangled leg, and that was pretty much that. So, that is how I found myself standing in theatre and, for the first time, operating on an animal I had genuine love for. I'm sure it will seem like something that must happen every week to a vet, but there was something special about this little guy. Sure we had had hundreds of stray animals in before and, yes, I often got attached to them, spending eleven or more hours a day with them, but any animal person will tell you, some are just extra special.

The decision was made to amputate the leg. The severity of the fractures meant that the surgery to fix the leg would be very advanced, with no guarantee of a good outcome. It would also cost the clinic a few thousand pounds, and as lovely as he was, unfortunately we couldn't justify spending so much money on a stray animal.

Writing it down it almost seems cold-hearted, just lopping off a leg, but if you have seen an animal on three legs it is a truly heartwarming sight. Amputation is generally avoided at all cost in humans – we see it as a bit of a failure when people need to have leg or arm amputations.

Generally it is a procedure reserved for those instances where there is simply no other option, or, Plan A has been tried and unfortunately failed. In animals, it's not that simple. I spend a large majority of my time around animals and I am regularly surprised at their tenacity and perseverance. They are fighters and survivors and I guarantee, if you give an animal three legs, they will get on with life like they know no differently.

Despite my hesitation at the start of surgery, once I made that first cut, I found my flow. It's odd, people ask me what it's like to operate. No matter whether it's a complex exploratory surgery or a simple routine procedure, I just seem to find a rhythm, as there is something almost harmonious about being in theatre.

When I was a student and then a newly qualified vet, I used to get really nervous. Nerves are good, they're there to make sure you don't fuck up from carelessness and they have saved my arse on a few occasions. When I first wanted to be a vet, I was really worried about surgery, not because it was hard, not because it was scary, but because of my tremor.

Since I was a teenager, I have had a little bit of an intention tremor, a mild shaking of my hands when I concentrate on something that requires heightened dexterity. Safe to say I was always crap at those ludicrously frustrating wire games where you have to get an electrified loop from one end of a wire to the other without setting off the buzzer. It isn't severe and by no means does it affect my day-to-day life, but when I was thinking about surgery and with nerves on top off that, it was a big concern of mine. I was lucky enough to see some practice in my local vet's at the age of sixteen and was watching a vet perform a cat spay. As I watched and chatted away with him, I kept noticing his hands making odd movements. His surgical skill was seamless, passing instruments and handling tissues as well as anyone I had ever seen, but every so often when he relaxed his hands, they started shaking violently. I asked him about it and he explained that he too had a tremor. I told him about my worries about surgery and he smiled. He had had exactly the same concerns, but it didn't seem to be causing him too much of an issue.

Eleven years later and I don't even think twice about it, and so, within fifteen minutes, I had the leg off, making my final cut through the femoral artery, which I had tied off to prevent the little guy bleeding out in front of me. The femoral artery is one of the biggest and most critical blood vessels in the body and I could feel myself holding my breath as I transected through it. There aren't many times I'll place two separate ligatures on a blood vessel, but the femoral artery is definitely one of them. It's a weird thing tying off and cutting through such a large blood vessel. You cut through it, your eyes fixed upon the remaining stump as it pulses along with the heart rate, watching for it to start pissing blood everywhere, which it inevitably does not.

'Now to close,' I said to my nurse.

'Make it neat,' she replied with a smile. That is the beauty of animals, they really don't care what they look like. Saying that, I really do and I take real care over the appearance of a wound. After all, it's the only bit of the operation you can see!

*

Half an hour later and I was sitting on the prep room floor, cradling my patient as he woke gently from his anaesthetic. It's not always a smooth process, but he couldn't have looked more adorable as he slowly blinked and licked his lips.

I often sit there watching animals coming round and wonder what must go through their minds. The last thing they must remember is being held by a nurse as a weird thing is put into their leg that stings a little sharply, then they start to feel all sleepy and suddenly they're waking up after an operation.

I'm sure there is a massive range of emotions as they come round – there certainly is in humans. Having spoken to some doctor friends of mine, there are patients that come round sleepily and smoothly, there are those that wake up entirely complimentary and lovey dovey (a bit like me when I had my appendix out) and then there are the thrashers, those people who become borderline dangerous and aggressive.

We deal with aggressive dogs regularly but there was one particular husky dog that I won't ever forget. It had been a proper pain in the arse trying to get him under anaesthetic. He had to be muzzled, which in itself was a palaver, and then he had fought us all the way, until he had finally succumbed to the 'sleepy juice' (Propofol is the real name, but I prefer 'sleepy juice'). It's well known that the dogs that go down fighting are generally the ones that throw themselves around on recovery too, but for whatever reason once the surgery was finished, he was left to be recovered by the smallest nurse in the practice; she was borderline 5ft tall and can't have weighed much more than about 6½ stone.

I heard it before I saw it. A crash came from theatre, and I spun on my heels and dived through the swinging doors. The dog had woken up with a start and thrown itself up into the air. The nurse had been doing her best to try to control him by literally throwing her whole weight on top of him, but it wasn't enough. As I came through the door she was flying backwards to my left, the dog having pushed her away with his front limbs. In doing so, he had thrown himself to my right, off the high surgery table and was heading towards the ground. Instinct took hold and I dived along the floor, spinning onto my back as I hit it, and skidded underneath the dog as he came down to land with a thump. I caught him, wrapped my arms around him and tried to calm him down. It was the single best catch I have ever made and every time I tell the story, people inevitably roll their eyes at me in response – I wish there had been a bloody camera in theatre.

In this little cat's case, if he had been a human I'm pretty sure he would have been confused and anxious, having lost a leg, but this little guy just lay there looking around, as if he

was seeing the room for the very first time. I sat there looking down at him and there and then made the decision to
take him home. The plan had been to do the op, get him
recovered and then either rehome him to a client of the
practice or send him on to Battersea Dogs and Cats Home.
But I just couldn't let him go. I was too invested, I had to go
all in. I had resisted this sort of temptation for years, but I
was destined to become one of the vets and vet nurses out
there with a pet they adopted from work. I told myself that
it was only going to be on trial basis as a 'foster' until he was
all healed and then I would see about finding him a perma-
nent home . . . yeah right. I called my sister and gave her the
news. She had already guessed this was coming, and even
managed to sound a bit excited about finally getting to meet
the cat she had heard so much about.

I finished work at eight that evening and jumped into the
shed to fish out a 'donated' cat carrier. Vet practices end up
as a bit of a dumping ground for surplus cat boxes and blankets and towels. Don't get me wrong – they're all hugely
useful, but there is something quite sad about taking a box
from someone, as they inevitably had a cat that recently
died or was put to sleep.

The box I picked had a piece of tape on the top of its plastic shell that simply read 'Geoff'. I wondered what happened
to Geoff and couldn't help but hope to myself that it was
nothing infectious. I made sure to give the box a thorough
clean with heavy duty disinfectant (just in case) and then
went to get my new pal. I bundled him up in a blanket and

plonked him into the carrier. He looked so small lying there with his wide eyes, and I wondered if he had any idea what was going on. I went through my mental check list: after all, I had nothing at home to cater for a pet cat. Pain relief, check, buster collar, check, litter tray, check, food, check.

'Okay then, little fella, looks like you're coming home with me,' I said through the carrier door. He stared back, and I knew he understood. I couldn't quite believe how chilled out he was. I placed him on the passenger seat of my car and we drove home together, listening to Ed Sheeran to keep my new three-legged flatmate calm on the journey. As we drove, I wondered if he had ever been in a car before or if he was confused to be inside one of the mechanical monsters he had the misfortune of being hit by some ten days ago? It was dark, rainy and cold, one of those October evenings that reminds you that winter is just around the corner. I covered the carrier, so he wouldn't get wet, and jumped out of the car, rushing him up to my flat.

I placed him on the floor and whipped the top off the carrier. He poked his head up like a meerkat and took in his surroundings. He popped out of the box, already elegant with his single hind limb, and made his way over to the sofa. He sniffed around and started to become acquainted with his new home. It took him all of five minutes to settle himself in, curling up in a ball on the sofa while I cooked dinner. 'I should probably give you a name, little guy,' I said to him. 'What do you reckon? Should we put it to the people?' I grabbed my phone and snapped a photo of him looking all adorable. I put it straight onto Instagram and within two hours I had a hundred name suggestions flying at me, my personal favourites being 'Captain Cat Sparrow' and 'Legoless', both appealing to my inner geek.

It was only later as my sister and I were watching television that I laughed to myself. 'Right, there is only one name for a three-legged black cat,' I said to Bethan. 'Say hello to Tripod.'

8

The Joys of Being a Vet

If you were to ask me to list my strengths in my job, I would probably put my consulting style pretty high up there. Some people would say I'm an extrovert and like nothing more than to engage people in conversation, while others might put it more bluntly and say I can talk the hind legs off a donkey. Either way, I pride myself on being able to read a situation and adjust as smoothly as a chameleon to anything that is thrown at me.

Everyone has an off day, though – right?

*

It had been a particularly long day. Multiple euthanasias followed by a ninety-minute enterotomy (surgery to open up the small intestine, in this case to remove a sock from a nine-month-old puppy) had left me sweaty, hungry and emotionally drained. I shovelled a questionable cheese sandwich down my neck too quickly, and went off to make a coffee before starting my afternoon consult block.

Having to jump from intense, high-pressure surgery to lighthearted consulting is a skill that takes time and practice to master. Only now, after five years of doing this every day, can I say I'm getting better at it, but by no means have I mastered it. I still sometimes look back at the first few consults of an evening and think, 'Wowee, people have come to see the professional vet, not a coked-up ADHD child.' You may laugh but that is genuinely how I can feel when I come out of these surgeries: high as a kite, followed by a massive crash back down to earth. My poor clients.

I looked at my list. 'Excellent,' I thought, as I saw that Steve was my first consult. Steve (that is the dog, not the owner) was in for a standard health check and, if I was lucky, I could get it out the way quickly and get back to my coffee and writing my surgical notes. Note writing is something you're not told about at university: it's the qualified vet's dirty little secret. You spend so much time working towards treating animals, you tend to overlook that a huge portion of your time as a vet is spent in front of a computer writing down what you have done and what you have observed in your patients, as well as replying to emails answering questions ranging from 'What food should I feed my puppy?' to 'Here is a picture of my cat's diarrhoea, what's she got?' Don't even get me started on the hours of phone calls.

I had met Steve once or twice before: he had been a strong-willed puppy, wriggling all over the place, making a simple clinical examination a fight and a half. He was only a small terrier, but he was strong as an ox, even as a pup. I read on through Steve's notes and my heart sank slightly. His behaviour had been getting worse each time he had come to the vet's, so much so that the last time he came he had been given the bitey crocodile symbol on his record. There are a number of symbols that you can put on an animal's account but the bitey crocodile is my favourite: both comical and fair warning. On the day that I was rushed and had a million other things to be doing, I would have bet my left testicle that Steve would make the appointment as difficult as possible. Oh, if only I had known.

I called Steve and his owner into my consult room through a forced toothy grin. Steve was a young Jack Russell Terrier, aged somewhere between one and two years. He was tricolour, with splodges of black, brown and white. He was a rather handsome dog, lean and muscly, with ears pricked, constantly at attention. He reminded me of one of my dogs, Jasper. We had picked up Jasper when I was in my early teens, a birthday present to my sister from my parents. Looking back now, we were silly really: he had been bred by some gypsies and despite that, we paid up and took him off them. I don't know whether it was due to a difficult start in life or something else but he turned out to be, for want of a better phrase, a little shit. Jack Russells can be difficult and I had first-hand experience of this.

'How's the little fella doing?' I asked Steve's owner cheerily.

'Oh, he's just wonderful, nothing to report. Just here to say hello and have a quick check over,' the owner replied.

'Excellent!' I exclaimed, bending down to Steve's level and offering a hand for him to have a sniff. This was test number one – I always start with a gentle, slow hello to all my patients unless I know them really well. I am lucky enough to have twenty minutes with most of my clients so I have the luxury of being able to spend the first five minutes of each consult putting both owner and pet at ease. I speak to colleagues within the veterinary industry about consulting times, and it wasn't that long ago that vets were still trying to stick to five minute consults and I'm sure there are some out there that still do. I've never understood how you can give a full consultation in five minutes; it often takes me that long just to welcome the owner in and say hello to the pet, let alone examine and treat the animal. If there are any vets reading this, I know they will be rather jealous and in mild disbelief that I get a full twenty minutes with each of my clients, and you better believe it's a much better way of life. I think sometimes as vets we underestimate how stressful it can be for an owner to come to the vet's, especially if they have a dog or cat that doesn't enjoy the experience. I regularly have to counsel owners through this as they feel utterly embarrassed at the behaviour of their pet.

I remember when I was a kid, my mother would put off taking the cats to the vet if she could. They hated getting into the carrier and she swears to this day, as do a lot of the owners I speak to, that cats are psychic and know when there is something awry. (I must add here that my mother is one hundred percent an animal lover and she would always take the cats to the vet's if they needed it – this avoidance was mainly just for routine checks.) The stress of putting a cat in a carrier and having them make a bid for freedom, shouting all the way to the vet's, or having to tell your little pup that you're going to the park and then see the realisation dawn on their face as you pull into the car park at the vet's, is enough to put anyone off wanting to come to the clinic. Steve had been one of those dogs, happy as little old Larry until his owner had taken the left at the end of the road, instead of the right towards the lovely hour-long walk they usually had around the common. I never like to see a dog dragged into the vet's but unfortunately that's how Steve's morning had gone.

Now Steve was in my consult room, and I sat across from him holding out a hand to say hello. He had clearly decided his time was better spent trying to scratch his way through the door that had closed behind him, the gateway to freedom, rather than engaging in any niceties. Realising that this tactic clearly wasn't working, I suggested that the owner pick him up and put him on the consult table. For me, this usually goes one of two ways. Sometimes it alerts the dog that it's business time and they need to sit and chill out while I do whatever I need to do. They get a treat and then they can go home. For others, it just adds height into the equation, presenting the owner with the challenge of keeping the dog on the table while it attempts to scale their shoulders. Steve decided he would sit and watch what was going on, taking everything in. I tried again to offer an olive branch (or a hand) and this time he was having none of it. His lip came up and he showed me exactly what he was thinking . . . as well as a lovely shining canine tooth.

I try not to make a habit of being bitten by my patients. Saying that, I never take it personally when an animal takes a disliking to me. That was particularly hard when I was first starting out as a vet. I had always been the animal lover – the person with a true affinity with animals – and then as soon as I became 'the vet' not every animal liked me quite as much. I am very lucky to have never been properly bitten by a patient. In fact, it was only this year that I got nipped for the first time. It was sort of a cross between a head-butt and a bite by a rescue Weimaraner dog. It was my own fault entirely and I was lucky that she just gave me a warning nip right on the bridge of my nose. Either way, getting bitten is never top of my to-do list.

I told the owner that Steve was giving me a warning, but she carried on obliviously chatting about her imminent holiday to Cyprus. I interrupted her, pointing out for a second time that Steve looked like he was going to try to bite me. She immediately took offence, 'Oh, my Stevie wouldn't do that, he loves everyone!' she said, cuddling her little pup into her bosom.

'Okay,' I said, and decided I would try one more time and give him a bit of a reassuring pat. I slid my hand across the table and to give him a bit of a rub on his bum. I had hardly touched him when he spun so quickly that I only just managed to retrieve my fingertips before his jaw clamped shut. He lunged again, just catching my retreating right hand. The owner gasped and responded by telling her darling pooch that it was 'all okay' and 'the nasty man isn't going to hurt you'. NASTY MAN?! I had hardly done anything, and her dog had just tried to take my hand off! I watched, a little rattled, as she reached into her designer handbag and pulled out a dog treat. Steve took it, looking very happy with himself. I am no canine behaviourist (something that is touched upon, though not in great detail at veterinary school), but even I can tell you this is not good dog training. What the owner had essentially done was tell Steve that the man across the table who he thinks is scary enough to warn off, is indeed very scary, and not only that, she has then rewarded his aggression with a yummy snack.

I quickly resisted the urge to explain this to the owner, convincing myself that it would probably fall on deaf ears right now and it would be better explained later on, once Steve was sufficiently far away from my fingers. A better use of my time, I thought, was to change tack and try with Steve on the floor. I asked the owner to take him back down from the table and took a handful of treats. I slowly encouraged Steve to come closer but, again, to no avail. He simply sat behind his mummy's legs and watched as a silly man (me) threw treats onto the floor and tried to mimic his owner's cooing phrases. Nope, this wasn't going to work.

The time had come to suggest to the owner that a 'party hat' (as we like to refer to muzzles in the veterinary industry) was not only going to be necessary here, but also beneficial to both the dog and me. I always offer to stop the consult in these instances, because bad experiences can actually just make the dog worse and worse until eventually there is simply no coming back from it. I've been quite lucky not to encounter that many dogs of this temperament, but I'm always very careful not to push them too far.

The owner had explained that she wanted me to check something on Steve's side, so in this case a muzzle was going to be necessary. Despite having just seen her puppy's inner wolf come to the surface, she was quite reluctant to agree to the muzzle, asking if I could just try again. But after that performance, I politely refused and suggested that if she wanted me to do anything with Steve beyond sitting on the floor for ten minutes trying to get him to take a treat from me, a muzzle was going to be needed. I could almost feel her roll her eyes as I turned and went to find a muzzle.

I came back and explained to the owner how to place it on Steve. I always suggest the owners do this, especially if the dog isn't used to wearing one, as the dogs generally mind it less if their trusted family member does it rather than me. Unfortunately, in this case, the owner couldn't quite grasp how the muzzle worked and asked if I could do it. I reluctantly obliged and having asked the owner to return Steve to the tabletop, tried to slip it over the dog's nose. Inevitably, he spun again, no doubt trying to take my arm off, snapping at the air around him. This time, though, I was ready and managed to catch hold of his harness, expertly spinning the sharp end away from me. I felt Steve tense up and pause in mid-air, ready to snap out at any of my appendages entering his peripheral vision. I stopped and took stock of the situation.

I had my right hand on Steve's harness, the muzzle in my left hand well away from his nose, and his front paws were pointed out, tense as anything, at the owner, his back legs planted on the table in front of me. I looked up at the owner, tears now streaming from her eyes: she was clearly not used to seeing this side of her darling little man. I must admit, even I was impressed at the swear words coming from Steve on this particular occasion – he was very unhappy about me being in his vicinity and he was letting me know about it. It can be really quite distressing seeing an ordinarily placid and happy little pooch turn into a savage beast in front of your eyes, but that is part and parcel of working with animals. A rare one, I'm pleased to add.

'What else can go wrong?' I thought to myself, as I tried and undoubtedly failed to explain to the owner that he was okay, I was not hurting him and this was something that we could work on. As I continued to assure her that he 'really isn't that bad and it isn't her fault', I became increasingly aware that something was awry. Steve had started to calm down and was now relaxing; his whole body had been as stiff as a board but now he was standing all fours on the consulting table and starting to look around. Maybe he had started to realise that the man standing behind him with his hand on his harness genuinely wasn't trying to kill him. He didn't even growl when I took a startled step back as the smell of faeces suddenly hit my nostrils. I loosened my grip on Steve's harness and looked down. I was greeted by a sight that I will never forget and that can only be described as 'poo-mageddon'. Not only had I earlier missed the fact that the owner had started crying, but I had also overlooked the liquid faecal matter that had been sprayed all over my front and shoes as I had so 'expertly' spun Steve away from me. I had been so concerned about the sharp front end of the dog that I had forgotten about Steve's explosive rear end. I picked Steve up – he didn't even bother reacting at this point, clearly aware that his job was done. I slowly placed him on the floor and he scampered away.

I think even Steve would have felt that, now I was covered in diarrhoea, I was less appealing as a chew toy and probably just someone to give a wide berth. I took a deep breath, which it turned out was not the thing to do when you've just been shat upon. I was now a walking turd, with a hint of anal gland. I hastily excused myself from the consult room and legged it to the prep area, the liquid faeces seeping through my clothing to my skin with every small movement. I started removing my clothes as soon as the consult room door swung closed behind me. I'm sure it's not something you're likely to wonder about, but imagine being diarrhoea-ed upon by a dog. Then imagine said diarrhoea seeping into your top and starting to cling to your midriff. Now imagine having to take that top off, over your head. As the top passed over my face I could have vomited. It wouldn't have mattered having another bodily fluid over my top. I threw the top in the sink and then dropped my trousers.

Inevitably, my nurse emerged from around the corner just at that point and got the shock of her life. It's fair to say you end up as a pretty close knit team working in veterinary. Rather than running in the other direction, she helped me by grabbing a bucket of water, some antiseptic wash and a towel. I sponged myself down, dried myself off and five minutes later I was safely back in a new set of scrubs. I gingerly returned to the scene of the crime. I hadn't really surveyed the scene in the consult room before leaving; I had been slightly preoccupied by the diarrhoea dripping from my scrubs. Incredibly, as it turned out, except for a little splash over the table, almost all of the diarrhoea had hit me and not the room. I began to clean down the table as the owner started on an apology. I cut her off, saying it was all okay and no harm done. But she interjected, 'No, no, I was just going to say . . . should we be worried about the colour of that diarrhoea? I'm worried Steve might be ill!'

I took a long chug of my coffee, and only after settling back in my chair realised that I hadn't checked the mug for faecal matter. I banished the thought and looked at the owner, then at Steve and then back at the owner. 'Honestly, I'm only really worried that it was down my front. If he carries on having diarrhoea then we can get him some treatment but let's see how he goes for now,' I said with a straight face. We chatted some more and I didn't touch Steve again. We settled on a plan of the owner going away and coming back in a few weeks once Steve had calmed down when we would see how we could go with a nice slow behaviour consult. I resisted the urge to remind the owner that only ten minutes before that I had suggested we just take it slow with Steve. I think she read from my face that I was likely to have a serious sense of humour failure if she asked me to look at the 'thing' on Steve's side again, so she tactfully let that one lie. Happy(ish) owner, happy(ish) dog, less happy vet. The owner turned to leave and I think even Steve was shocked that he had managed to get away without so much as an exam. As the owner said her goodbye and walked through the consult door I watched in disbelief as Steve cocked his leg and pissed up the door frame. I'm not sure if it's my memory playing tricks on me, but I'm convinced he winked at me over his shoulder as he strutted away.

I was in the pub a few weeks later with a vet friend of mine. As much as we try, when vets get together we cannot help but talk about work. I'm sure it's the same with all friends in similar industries. At uni we used to take the piss out of people for only being able to talk about animals and veterinary even in the most unlikely of places. I'm not exaggerating when I tell you I was once in the middle of the dance floor in a central London night club, dancing with another vet student, when she leaned over to me and asked, 'What's the cutest patient you had this week?' Dear Christ.

Either way, I was recounting this tale to my friend and after taking an inordinate amount of time to hide his amusement (which he utterly failed to do), he said to me, 'So let me get this straight. The dog bit you, the owner cried, you got shat on AND he pissed up the wall?'

'Yuhuh,' I replied, with a strange admiration for the little dog.

'Mate, that's the quadfecta!' And so it became known amongst my friends as the 'quadfecta', the absolute worst possible combination of things to happen in a consult. That is what you call an epic fail.

*

One of the things I love the most about the veterinary profession is the closeness of a veterinary team. I work with some of the best people I know, I trust them absolutely and I know they have my back. I don't know if I have just been lucky, but I have always found that vets and nurses alike have a very special bond. Some might think too close a bond – I would love to know the official percentage of vets dating vets or vet nurses: I guarantee you it's higher than you think. Some of my best friends are vets, none more so than Rose. Rose and I became friends at university. We revised together for exams, we were emotional crutches for each other through the highs and lows of vet school and then we ended up working together in our first job. While I worked nights and emergency shifts, she was at one of the branches and still works there to this day.

When I left that job, we kept in touch and we meet regularly for a drink and a catch-up, getting up to date with all the gossip from my old colleagues. We were having a coffee recently and I was asking about the new emergency team. I must admit I can't help but compare myself to the people working my old job. I like to think I am pretty good at my job so I slightly revel in the thought that my old boss would want me to go back and work there. As I asked, Rose couldn't help herself, 'Oh my God you're going to love this one,' she started, and so the story began.

She had been starting her morning shift and went in for handover, essentially a walk around the hospital to discuss and hand over the patients from overnight to the day vet. It had been a new night vet on – Rose thought she was from Romania and a really nice woman. She had been doing nights a while, she was pretty switched on and so they started going through the handover. She went to the dog ward where she had a patient in with HGE (haemorrhagic gastroenteritis, aka, very serious shits), fine, a dog that had been hit by a car, fine. So they went to the cat ward: a diabetic cat, one boarding post-surgery, and another – Rose couldn't actually remember what it was in for. They had headed back to the prep room and were just chatting when the lovely Romanian vet said, 'Hey, sorry, I forgot to tell you about the other thing I have in. It was brought in by a guy last night – I think it might have been hit by a car. I've never really seen one before but I had a google and I think it's a giant wild ferret . . .' At this point I was taking a sip of my coffee and I spurted it out my nose. 'A GIANT WILD FERRET? What on earth did she have in?!' I laughed to Rose.

'Oh just you wait . . .' she replied.

Rose had managed to hold her amusement in better than I did, humoured her and asked her what this 'giant wild ferret' had been like. She said, 'Well, at first it was a bit sedated, so I gave it some pain relief, then once it started to feel better it was an aggressive fucker so I had to muzzle it to examine it. I think it's fine but it might be worth X-raying to be sure.' So Rose asked to see it. They took a walk upstairs to the exotics ward, a small box room with a number of vivariums and heated kennels mainly for patients with feathers or scales. In the middle of the room there was a pop-up cage with a large blanket over the top. The Romanian vet grabbed a corner of the blanket and threw it back to reveal the giant wild ferret, or, as Rose told her through tears of laughter, a badger. Apparently they don't have badgers in Romania.

I laughed at that story for a full five minutes. I missed working with Rose. We always had a laugh, but when we worked together we also made each other better vets. We had a friendly competitive edge, but also worked well together. In fact, the whole team had worked well together, which was a good thing when the surgery got an emergency call one summer morning. The call was from a member of the public. They had been in the park walking their dog when they had seen a dog walker struggling with a number of dogs from across the park. She had walked over and, as she had neared, realised that the struggle was in fact full-on panic. The dog walker was dragging one young dog out of the park's 'pond', surrounded by about ten dogs in total. One by one, as if they had all been put under some sort of spell, the dogs had started vomiting. She had helped the dog walker load the dogs into her car and was calling to let us know she was on her way to us. Ten vomiting dogs, all at once.

Something wasn't right. We had seven vets at the hospital that day, and a good thing too. Ten vomiting dogs, though – surely one or two vets could handle that, no big deal. Wrong. By the time the dogs arrived, the dog walker was in floods of tears: as she had been driving, some of the dogs had been getting worse – they had started collapsing and some even started to have seizures. This had just gone from DEFCON 4 to DEFCON 1. The receptionist hit the tannoy and half shouted 'Code red reception, all vets to reception, I repeat CODE RED!' We spilled out of the break room, out of the prep area, out of consults and suddenly seven vets all descended on the poor dog walker. She pointed us to her car and we ran out to grab the dogs. Some were seizuring, some were covered in their own vomit, some couldn't hold their own weight. We carried them into the prep area and started working on them as quickly as we could. Ten dogs, seven vets and an amazing team of vet nurses. I had never been a part of something like this and I don't think I will ever be part of something like it again.

For the few weeks leading up to this, it had been unseasonably warm weather. This increase in temperature accompanied by other rather specific conditions had allowed for an environmental phenomenon known as an algal bloom. The particulate algae that had multiplied in its millions over a period of forty-eight hours was one of the blue-green variety, and, more importantly, one that is highly toxic to dogs. The poor dog walker wasn't aware of this and had encouraged the dogs under her care to go and cool off in the park's pond. The dogs had obliged and dived in head first, and that was all it took. In a few minutes they were all starting to succumb to the toxic effects of the little plant. The clinical signs of algal poisoning in dogs include vomiting, diarrhoea, collapse, seizuring and, in severe cases, death.

I was working on one of the less severe dogs – he was vomiting and panting but he was conscious and had no signs of any neurological abnormalities. I worked with a nurse to place an intravenous catheter and started the dog on a high rate of fluids, trying to prevent any further signs. I looked around – the room was mayhem, and there were vets and nurses running around trying to save the lives of more animals than we had tables. I suddenly saw one of the other vets shout – I couldn't quite hear her over the din but I could tell from her eyes that it wasn't good. My dog was doing okay so I ran over to her; the dog had crashed and she had started compressions, trying to bring him back. I looked down at young Golden Retriever that she was trying to save. We alternated doing compressions for ten minutes.

When you watch people do CPR on television, they are far too gentle. The first time I ever had to do compressions was on a large Labrador and the vet I was working with at the time had given me one piece of advice: 'Don't fuck around, break some ribs.' It may sound brutal but he isn't totally wrong, you really do have to put your back in to it, hence the two of us sharing the load. As I traded out of compressions after about two minutes, I looked around. I had been caught up in the puppy we were working on and everything else in the room had sort of faded into the background. As I looked, I saw four other vets doing CPR. Five of the dogs were dying – it was a nightmare. There is no concept of time in those situations. Your entire focus is on the life in front of you and how you're going to save it. A very rare sequence of events had led to our team of vets all working in harmony, trying to save the lives of ten dogs.

Three dogs died, despite our efforts. Seven survived. Without the work of the incredible vets and nurses on that day, more lives would definitely have been lost. Working at a hospital can be intense, hard work, but on days like that you feel like you're a part of something incredible. Vets around the country are doing amazing work, but there aren't many practices that could have dealt with such a large number of dogs in an emergency situation like that one.

Vets really need to support each other. High-pressure, emotional situations can be incredibly draining and take a huge amount out of you. It took the whole team a while to get over that day and we were still reeling from it a few weeks down the line. Everyone had been a little overwhelmed by the whole ordeal, but the outcome had been seven dogs had gone home back to their owners. I'm not sure many of us could have expected more.

9

When It All Gets Too Much

It may not surprise you to learn that there is a huge mental health issue in the veterinary profession, the extent of which is only just now coming to the fore. It is well documented that approximately one in four people in the general population will face a mental health issue each year, but early figures suggest much, much higher rates in vets.* One horrifying statistic is that vets are four times as likely to commit suicide as the general public – that's twice as likely as doctors and dentists. As a profession, we regularly come right at the top of suicide risk lists. Vetlife charity reports evidence of increased psychological distress in the veterinary profession when compared to others, with higher levels of anxiety, depressive symptoms, suicidal thoughts and suicide risk. In recent years, and with statistics as shocking as these, the mental health crisis within the veterinary profession has started to come to the forefront, with charities such as Vetlife leading the way in aiding those who are struggling. As with any mental health issue, it has been a slightly taboo

* (https://www.vetlife.org.uk/mental-health/depression; Platt et al 2010)

subject for far too long a time. I have tried over the last few years to start having the conversation and discussing the toll of the job with anyone who would listen. It's not uncommon for others within the profession to shy away at first, but once I talk about my own experiences and the things I struggle with, they often open up about their issues as well. Almost every single vet I speak to has their own story or their own negative feelings that they deal with on a regular basis.

I have always been an open person: I don't deal well with hiding my feelings. As much as I try, and believe me I do, I just cannot suppress emotion – it bubbles up and either comes out as rage or sadness. I had my share of issues at university, including a particularly bad year that threw me into a downward spiral which ended up with me failing a year. Don't get me wrong, I'm sure no-one has a completely smooth ride through university, but I struggled with the transition from school to uni life. Being a sheltered Cotswolds boy, uprooted and thrown headfirst into a central London university experience was a lot, to say the least. Despite a pretty rubbish year, I have always been a strong believer that I can pick myself up and get on with the job, and at the time that is exactly what I did. I had never really quite grasped what it was to be depressed; I was very lucky in my family, my friends and my career, so much so that I didn't feel like I could be depressed. That is, until a week back in 2017 that pushed my already fragile, hugely stressed self over the edge into a pit of negativity that even I couldn't break out of without asking for help. This is how it went.

*

The weekend had been filled with the usual self-medication of alcohol and late nights out in some nameless, sticky-floored London bar, followed by a Sunday in bed with fried chicken and copious amounts of coffee. This had become an all too common waste of a weekend, not looking after myself at all. On the Monday I had come in to meet my first patient of the day, a cat that had seen one of my colleagues over the weekend while I was no doubt two pints deep. It was old, skinny and clearly not in a great way but the most friendly little thing. The owners were a kind and smiley couple, the Kims. They had seen the cat coming into their garden for a few months, getting progressively skinnier and skinnier, eventually to the point that they were worried the cat was ill. They had started putting food out for it a few weeks after seeing it, which it had eaten with gusto. They had finally caved, feeling so sorry for the poor cat that they had brought him into the clinic for a check-over to see if, firstly, he had an owner, and, secondly, he was in decent health. My colleague had scanned him for a microchip, but he didn't have one. The Kims had been posting on social media for weeks, checking all the normal places for lost cats on Facebook and Twitter pages. They had had no luck, so it looked like he was homeless and a stray. My colleague had talked to the couple and they decided, having not wanted a cat, that they would take him on as their own and make sure he got a good life. When this sort of thing happens, it makes my heart sing with joy at the kindness of humanity. These people could so easily have dropped the cat off in a box at any vet's or rescue centre and forgotten all about him, but no, there was something inherently good inside them that made them want to help.

Now to address his health. He was clearly an older cat, though probably looked older than he actually was. He had been losing weight which was clearly now of concern, and recently, despite putting out his favourite Whiskas food (don't worry we got them to upgrade that pretty sharpish), he had been turning his nose up at all tasty treats for a few days, likely contributing to his now quite marked weight loss. My colleague had written notes of what she had found over the weekend – nothing obvious but concerns over a few possible underlying issues. She had given the cat some medications to try to help his appetite, and told them to have a discussion about whether they were going to keep the cat on and pay for further investigations. She had outlined the costs, with significant discounts based upon the situation, and booked them in to see me once they were sure that they were going to take him on.

*

The couple came in with their new cat that morning in his fancy new carrier and proudly announced that they were going to take 'Aslan' on for good. I knew they wanted the best for him. 'Ahh, you guys are amazing, and what an awesome name! I love C.S. Lewis,' I said, as they told me their decision. I was delighted and warmed to the couple immediately – they had something about them that I couldn't help but succumb to: Aslan had lucked out. After chatting some more with the Kims, they told me that they didn't have children and I think they were seeing this as their duty to help an innocent animal, as if he had chosen them. They must have been coming to retirement age and I wondered to myself if this was their way of starting a little family. What a wonderful fairytale this was turning out to be.

We needed to do some blood work on Aslan since, as happy as the couple were to have him in their lives, he wasn't a well cat. He still hadn't eaten over the weekend and today he was starting to look a bit sick, more lethargic and his eyes had lost their sparkle. I examined him as the couple looked on and cooed over their newly adopted family member. There was a bit of a bad smell hanging around Aslan; he definitely wasn't living up to his regal namesake. He was all skin and bones, his eyes slightly sinking into his skull, making him look about my age (which is like 200 for a cat). As I looked down at him he mewed at me, his mouth open wide and, just like that, I knew where the smell was coming from. His breath was as though it had been emitted from Satan's bottom (as my mother would say). If there had been a bunch of flowers in the room they would have wilted. Aslan's teeth were terrible – maybe that's why he had gone off his food? I suggested to his owners that the blood work should be followed by a general anaesthetic to address those horrendous teeth. I offered them a 50 percent discount as a gesture of goodwill. It's really hard in these situations: a few days before, the couple had no pets and no financial responsibility for any animals, but now this little guy had walked into their lives and they were being quoted a large sum of money for vital dental work. They were thankful for the offer of a discount, but I again reiterated to them that we could probably find a place for Aslan at a charity that would do this work for him. They declined and said that they felt he had found them for a reason, and it was their duty to help. God, I loved that couple.

Aslan spent the day with me. His bloods were normal except for some mild dehydration, which was the best news, and we quickly moved onto addressing the cesspit he called a mouth. It's rare that I'm squeamish with smells, but even I made sure to wear gloves and a mask while dealing with Aslan. I'm not sure I've met many living creatures that smelt so close to a rotting corpse. 'I've dissected bodies that smelt better than you, mate,' I said to him as I induced his anaesthetic. He drifted off to sleep and I placed a tube into his throat, all the while trying to stay as far away from his mouth as possible. I knew Aslan's mouth was going to be a bit of a shit show from the smell of it, but I'm not sure I was quite prepared for what lay ahead of me. I started removing teeth, one after the other, and when I say removed, I mean pulled out with my fingers.

Dentistry is not one of the things I love about my job, in fact if you were to ask any nurse or vet I've worked with over the years what my least favourite part of the job is, I'm pretty sure every single one would give you the correct answer of dentistry. In vet practices across the country, you will find vets working away on the mouths of pets. It is rarely delicate, it is rarely intricate and, at least when I perform dental surgery, it is generally accompanied by a stream of profanities and sweat. I will never understand how some teeth manage to attach themselves so solidly into the skull of an animal. It is with those thoughts in mind, then, that when I tell you I removed TWENTY teeth from this cat's mouth, and I repeat, without using any instruments, and the fact that I was finished in less than fifteen minutes, you may be able to appreciate how diseased this guy's teeth were. No wonder the wee fella wasn't eating. How could he? The only positive to his mouth being so bad was the speed at which I could work and remove the rotten teeth from his skull. I had him fixed up in no time, pain medications on board, and he soon recovered from his anaesthetic and started taking his course of antibiotics.

He really was a sweet little cat and I sat with him while he recovered. Soon enough, he was up, head-butting my hand for a bit of extra love. I must admit I didn't expect much when I went to offer him some soft food – after all his mouth must have been terribly uncomfortable – but I could barely believe my eyes as he threw himself head first into the food bowl, almost knocking it out of my hand with his eagerness. It's times like that when I feel like we are making a real difference to animals. He had come in that morning off his food with a horrendously painful mouth and now he was tucking into his second large bowl of meaty goodness. I called the Kims and gave them the good news, something that rarely loses its novelty, and Aslan went home that night to his happy new owners. Monday was a good day, and I drove home that evening with a smile on my face, my hangover from the weekend having faded into the past.

*

Tuesday. This was a relatively quiet day: I spent the morning revelling in the glow from the day before, seeing a number of consults. The highlight was a consult with a lady and her new Golden Retriever puppy. She was really quite attractive and the puppy was darn right gorgeous so I was on the charm offensive from the get-go. My general approach with new clients was to try to make them and their pets feel as comfortable as possible on their first visit, making them both want to come back, not dread it. As vets we have a tendency to underestimate how stressful it can be coming into the clinic, so I have made it my mission to make the experience as enjoyable as possible with plenty of cups of tea or coffee for the clients and all the treats for the patients.

I spent the full forty minutes cooing over the puppy while

asking the owner all the standard questions such as 'What is he eating?' and 'Where did you get him from?' The owner was sweet but it was clear from the outset that she hadn't really had dogs before, and research wasn't something she had time for before getting the puppy. I patiently gave her my advice on a wide range of things, suggesting she wrote notes so that she had a record for reference.

The one thing that the owner was adamant about was vaccinations: 'I don't want to vaccinate him,' she kept repeating. I tried to start to explain the benefits of vaccination and the reasons we did this but she was having none of it. 'It's just not necessary,' she started, 'I just haven't seen him be even the slightest bit nasty to anyone,' she carried on.

Had I missed something? I thought to myself. Why was she suddenly talking about his temperament? 'Wait, sorry, what does his behaviour have to do with vaccination?' I asked her, trying to hide my frustration.

'Well, my friend told me about the distemper vaccination and I just don't think it's necessary. Do all dogs have it?' I must have looked like she was speaking Klingon as she didn't wait for my reply. 'I just don't think he has a bad temper so why does he need dis-temper?'

I burst into laughter. I really should have been more professional but I couldn't help it. She was shocked, clearly not expecting my outburst, and looked quizzically at me.

'Did one of your friends tell you it was a vaccination for his behaviour?' I asked, trying to offer her a way out of her faux pas.

'Well, is it not?' She said with mild disbelief. I smiled at her and explained that distemper was in fact a very serious viral infection in dogs and not a dog in a bad mood. I like to think her friend set her up for that one but, to this day, I'm not entirely sure that it wasn't just an innocent mistake. I maybe got more of a clue as we moved on from the vaccination chat to the puppy's weight and, as I tried to explain to her that he was just skinny because he was a puppy, she chimed in saying that when she picked him up she was really worried he was emancipated. I didn't bother to correct her.

The afternoon consisted of some routine surgery, some calls to clients, replying to some emails and a full reorganisation of the pharmacy. My first client of the afternoon was new to us, never been seen before, and I called the gentleman in with a smile on my face. He trundled into the room and I introduced myself. He wasn't the most forthcoming in his reply but I carried on, and started to get his cat out of its carrier. 'His skin is bad,' the owner offered up. Sometimes taking a history is like getting blood from a stone. I was slightly taken aback as I pulled the cat out further: he looked remarkably normal as I pulled his front out but as he emerged, his back end was almost completely bald, as if he was a sphinx cat. He most definitely was not, however; he was just a normal, short-haired cat, with very little hair from his belly button backwards. As I moved my hands over the skin, I could see the cat was incredibly itchy – his skin was writhing as I touched him. I manoeuvred him to get a good look at the extent of the damage. He was clearly so itchy that he had pulled a huge amount of his hair out and was now intent on scratching and chewing himself until he had made himself scabby and sore.

I'll never forget one of my dermatology professors at university – a Scot through and through, with an accent to match. He had given our skin lectures and, as it turned out, he was the specialist I was to report to when I was on my dermatology rotation. We had been looking at one of his cases, a cat, not too dissimilar to the one I was seeing that day, with a huge amount of hair loss. I had been putting together a list of differential diagnoses and had come up with a few serious conditions such as pemphigus and cutaneous lymphoma. The prof turned to me as I told him what I thought and said, 'You have to remember, Rory, cats are the self-harmers of the animal world and they will make everything look a lot worse than it is.'

In terms of skin disease, I think he is right, and I heard his Scottish voice playing through my head as I looked over the balding cat in front of me. It turned out, as I drew out more from the owner, that the cat was fifteen. He had been rescued two years previously and the skin had been this bad for somewhere between three and twelve months – the owner could not (or would not) remember. It can be very difficult to be impartial in these instances, as I have a duty to animals to be a guardian of their welfare. It is very easy when presented with cases like this to make snap judgements, but as a vet it is important not to judge owners too quickly. I was really struggling to get past this one though, as this guy had sat at home watching his cat eat away at himself for the last few months and done nothing about it. Ah, but he hadn't done nothing, he told me, he had bought some flea treatment from Sainsbury's and put that on him. He wasn't really sure if it had worked. I suggested gently that it clearly hadn't helped, pointing out the extent of the damage on the cat in front of me. I combed through the cat's remaining hair and just as I expected, found a large amount of flea dirt.

Flea dirt just looks like black dirt – it clogs up in a comb and you can tell it's flea poo by adding it to a small amount of water. It's quite a cool basic test. Fleas eat blood, so when you watch the black specks in water, they bleed and turn the water red. I did this with the owner, explaining that was the cause and was about to suggest a treatment plan when he said, 'Right, so it's not fleas because I've treated him. I had a bit of a google and I think it must be some sort of skin cancer so I think it's best we put him to sleep.' He said it with a straight face, looking almost annoyed that I hadn't come to the obvious conclusion myself. Throughout the consult, the gentleman across from me had been disconnected and monosyllabic, and it was like a switch had flicked. He had suddenly booted up and remembered what he was here to say. I was taken aback, half wondering if he was joking. This was most definitely a flea infestation, and even if it wasn't, the fleas were certainly contributing and could be very easily treated.

'I really don't think this is anything more serious than fleas,' I started, trying to help the owner see this was something we could treat. 'If this was cancer, I would expect some other signs.'

He looked at me, and plainly replied, 'I'm afraid I can't afford your expensive treatments, I think we should put him to sleep.' I was clearly not getting through to the owner and I became convinced there was something else going on. Something just didn't add up. I spent the following fifteen minutes going back and forth with the owner, pleading with him to allow me to treat the cat for flea infestation. The owner kept coming back to the same question: 'Can you promise me it's not something more than fleas?'

Obviously, I couldn't. Clients love to ask the hard questions such as 'What would you do?' or 'But if she was your cat . . .' I usually tried to give my best politician impression and answer the question by asking another question, or simply ignoring it and going off on a tangent. Unfortunately there was no getting away from it in this instance. I eventually used the last weapon I had left in my arsenal. I had pleaded, I had begged, I had offered a discount that would've made my boss blanch. The owner had taken none of it, insisting that the fairest thing to do was to end the cat's life. I simply couldn't do it.

'One last try,' I thought to myself as I geared up to play my final card. 'How about you sign your cat over to me so I can keep him here and try to treat him?' I asked, explaining that it would mean that he lost all rights to ownership of the cat, and that I would be responsible for its care, treatment, cost and finding it a new home. He looked plainly at me and for a minute I seriously thought he was going to attack me. Looking him dead in the eyes, I added, 'Please?'

'Okay,' he said. 'But I would much rather have him put to sleep . . .' he started.

I cut him off: 'Thank you so much.'

I quickly mocked up a form on the computer, ridding the owner of any responsibility, legal or financial and almost threw a pen at him I was so eager to get him to sign before he changed his mind. I watched with my heart in my mouth as he finally signed the form and looked up at me. 'It's not fleas,' he said again in a low voice and looked at me as if willing me to finally agree with him now the saga was over. I didn't, and told him to call if he needed anything; he turned and walked out the consult room door without looking back. I scooped up the cat, popped him in our biggest kennel and set him up with a litter tray and some food. He almost had my hand off as I was putting the food in, so I popped a worming tablet and some flea treatment in with the rest of the pouch of food, which he willingly swallowed down in a matter of moments. I watched him as he settled into his new kennel, having a sniff around, stopping every few seconds to give himself a scratch where his skin was itchy.

I called him Scratchy.

*

Wednesday. I could tell something was wrong as I pulled up at work. Mr Kim, Aslan's owner, was waiting for me at the door of the surgery. We opened at 8am and it was only 7:45. I walked up to him, concerned for Aslan. Had there been a problem after the op? Did he have a bad reaction to the drugs? Had he passed away from the anaesthetic? 'I don't know what to do, Rory . . .' the man said as I approached. He explained that Aslan was doing amazingly: he had a new lease of life since the surgery and had hardly stopped eating over the last few days. The problem was that Aslan's original owner had knocked on their door yesterday, asking for his cat back, finally having come across one of the Kims' Facebook posts from almost a month previously. I ushered the owner inside and made him a cup of tea. Consults didn't start until 8:20, so we sat in the waiting room and chatted.

'The thing is,' he explained, 'we spent about five hundred pounds on treating Aslan, and my wife is so in love with him, it just seems unfair.'

I had a horrible feeling in the pit of my stomach. I hate confrontation and I sensed that this wasn't going to come to an easy resolution. We discussed it further and agreed that when he saw the original owner he would ask for some financial compensation for the cost of the treatment we carried out on Monday.

After all, it was his cat and if he was going to take him back, it was the least he could do. I think we both knew it wasn't the last I would be seeing of Aslan and his owners when I waved him off that morning.

It was 11:15 and I had just finished my consults as I heard the bell ring from the front door of the clinic. Every time I had heard it go that morning I had hoped it wasn't Aslan's owners. I just wanted it all to be resolved and Aslan to be happy. I told you I hate conflict, right? There were no more consults booked for the morning so I wandered into the reception area with the pretence of getting a coffee. There was a man at the desk speaking to the receptionist – he was about 5ft 6in tall and wiry in stature. He was wearing a white T-shirt with paint all over it, and blue jeans with similar paint splatters, clearly a tradesman or a keen DIY enthusiast. I went over to the coffee station and boiled the kettle, trying to listen in to the conversation, but he had stopped talking as I had walked out.

'Are you the vet, pal?' He addressed me, almost spitting the words out, dripping in distaste.

'Yes, I am, can I help?' I said in a light tone, hoping the man was not who I thought he was. As I turned towards him, I knew exactly who he was. Aslan's new owner had given me a bit of a description that morning – this was clearly his previous owner.

'You owe me five hundred quid, mate,' said the man.

'I owe you what?' I asked, feigning ignorance to the situation. 'Sorry, I'm not sure I understand.'

'You saw my cat on Monday and you did a load of expensive tests and stuff that he didn't need and fleeced the guy that brought him in for five hundred quid; now he wants me to pay because it's my cat, so you owe me five hundred quid,' he said. He was edging closer to me as he talked, and I was starting to feel uneasy. His body language was aggressive and he was clenching his fists like he was going to hit out at any minute. As I've mentioned, I'm not really one for confrontation, and this man didn't seem like the kind of chap I could talk to reasonably.

'Right, okay, I think I know the cat you're talking about. The couple that brought him in told me he had been hanging around for a few months and he was really not in a good way when I saw him. I assure you that I wouldn't have done anything for the cat that was unnecessary.'

He didn't like that and stepped towards me. 'Don't give me that bullshit. All you vets are the same – charging people stupid money for things they don't need. I thought you were meant to like animals not use them to pay for your new car.' He had raised his voice and I instinctively took a step back. I turned and placed my coffee down. I could feel myself shaking and an anger was bubbling up inside me. Of course I had had people accuse me of charging too much – it was part and parcel of being a vet – but I had never been accused of making up illnesses and carrying out unnecessary procedures on animals. I had never been in a situation like this before. I felt genuinely threatened and I didn't know how to deal with it. I took a deep breath and faced the man; as I started speaking I wasn't really sure how it would go, but I had sort of come to terms with the fact that he may punch me for what I was about to say.

'Firstly, if you want to take that tone, I'm afraid you're going to have to leave. I will simply not have you speak to me or any of the staff here like that.' He tried to start but I held a hand up and continued to speak.

'Secondly, I can assure you, I am not in this job for the money, or in fact in the business of swindling people out of large sums of money for illnesses I happen to say their animals have. No vet I know enters into this job for the money – vets simply do not earn enough to allow for that. I am in this job because I love animals and want to help them in any way I can. Now, unfortunately, we are a business not a charity so we must charge for the service we provide, but by no means do we overcharge or do things that are unnecessary to inflate a bill. In fact, we often cut costs where we can and give as much discount to owners as we can afford. In your instance, I'm afraid this is a really tough situation.

'Your cat was, as I have been told, hanging around the garden of the lovely couple that brought him to me on Monday for the last few months. The cat had lost a lot of weight and looked very unwell, and they felt that they could no longer watch the cat suffer, so started feeding it, put up posters and put photos of him on social media, all of which, I'm afraid, you either did not see or did not respond to. They then reached the point where they were so worried that they brought him into us. At bare minimum, the cat had a severe and painful dental disease which needed fixing to keep him eating but also to stop him being in chronic pain. He was also very skinny and dehydrated. Obviously we checked our system for cats reported lost. Did you report him lost, by the way?'

The man seemed to be caught slightly unawares by my mid-rant question. I paused for an answer that did not come, and carried on.

'Right, so we also checked him for a microchip, which he didn't have. We explained to the couple that it was up to them what they did. They could either leave the cat with us and we would contact the RSPCA or they could take him on, which they chose to do. On Monday I ran blood tests, treated his dehydration and fixed his awful teeth, which clearly had been a problem for years, not just the last few weeks. At no point have I done anything unnecessary and your cat is now pain-free and happy. So, Sir, I would appreciate it if you didn't accuse me of mistreating animals or fleecing their owners as, at every point, I have done exactly what I thought right for your cat. What I suggest you do is come to an agreement with your cat's new owners as to whether you cover the cost of treatment, without which he would be suffering, or you allow them to take your cat and give him the loving home I know they can provide him.'

I stopped and took a breath, suddenly very aware of how much I was waving my arms around. My friends have always made fun of the fact that whenever I get passionate about something my arms and hands start to flail as if to try to back up my points. At that precise moment I was aware that I may have been slightly 'flaily' and didn't want to come across the least bit aggressive for the sake of my nose, so I gently lowered my arms to my side and awaited a response. I was shaking. I didn't really know what had come over me.

Clearly there was pent-up frustration that had been there for months, maybe years, which had all just come to the fore.

The man looked me up and down like I was a crazy person. My receptionist had stood up behind the desk and had a look on her face that was mainly disbelief, but with a hint of pride in there too. It was as if that moment froze in time: what can only have been a few seconds felt like it lasted a few minutes, and I started to wonder if the man was going to come at me again or if he would back down after my monologue. He did the latter, dismissing me by telling me to get my boss to call him, as he grabbed a pen from the reception desk and wrote down his name and number for me to pass on. I stood there like a lemon and took the piece of paper from him before he swung open the door of the clinic and left. I felt the adrenaline start to dissipate as soon as he was gone, and a wave of nausea came in its place. I was an odd combination of embarrassed and upset. I couldn't explain it – I had stood up to a bully; I should have felt invigorated and proud.

As the day went on I couldn't shake the embarrassment. It was as if the whole experience had rekindled a feeling I used to get when picked on at school, a feeling I hadn't had in more than ten years. I urged the day to move quickly but it dragged on. Even my favourite pair of dogs coming in couldn't break the funk I was in. They bounded into the practice as they always did, almost bowling me over in their enthusiasm and then jumped all over me, licking my face.

They are the happiest dogs, but even as they left I felt the mist descending again.

The day finally came to a close and I got into my car to drive home. I sat there and thought about Aslan and how lovely he was. I thought about the Kims and how lovely they were, how happy they had been to finally have a pet to dote on. I was sure the couple would give an amazing home to Aslan, but then there was his owner. I suddenly hated the man who had come into the clinic that day. I hated how he had made me feel, how he had made me doubt myself and feel misplaced guilt, like I had actually done something wrong. That's what I was feeling – I was doubting every decision I had made as a vet and all because an aggressive man had come into my work and threatened me and suggested that I was a bad person.

I sat there for ten minutes, tears running down my face and dripping from my chin. I felt broken and ashamed, but for no good reason. When I finally managed to pull myself together, I started the engine and drove home. I got home at eight o'clock and got straight into bed. I didn't eat dinner: I had no appetite. I fell asleep confused and concerned about my life choices. Had I got it all wrong?

*

Thursday. This was my day off and I woke early and lay there trying to process what had happened the day before. I was still questioning everything. I couldn't shake it. People had told me I wasn't good enough to be a vet before – were they right? I had failed some exams through uni. I had passed them second time round and I thought I had moved on from that but even then, lying in bed, the feelings of inadequacy that I had at that time came back. Had my failing those exams been some divine sign saying I wasn't cut out to be a vet? I thought back to Monday: I had done as much as I could to try to help with Aslan. I had spent Monday working to make him feel better and it sounded from Mr Kim as if he was a much happier cat since. I had given hefty discounts on the cost of the treatment, discounts that had landed me an email from my boss warning me that I was pushing the boundaries. My boss was great; she allowed me to make decisions in situations like this, and, pretty much, as long as I didn't take the piss, she let me get on with it – but even she had been irked by the level of discount I had thrown at the Kims. In trying to help an animal and his new owners, I had got myself in trouble at work. Fine, that I could deal with. I wasn't looking for a medal, I wasn't looking for appreciation, I knew how much it had meant to the Kims and they had been hugely grateful. But then to be threatened and my intentions questioned by an aggressive client? No. That was just not fair, and now the Kims were upset, my boss was annoyed and Aslan was probably going to end up back with an owner who didn't give a shit. I couldn't stop berating myself and questioning where I had gone wrong. I had questioned myself before, not quite like this but to a milder extent. Ordinarily I am a talker. My mum always says, 'If I hear from you, I know you're okay. It's when you don't call me that I know something's wrong.' And she is right. When I am mentally well, I talk to people. Particularly my mum and my dad. I tell them everything and they are my strongest of rocks. As I mentioned, I have always had great colleagues, and good friendships with my fellow vets and vet nurses. It's easy to say now, but I should have reached out. If there is anyone that understands these feelings as much as me, it's my colleagues. The emotional and mental toll of being a vet is something that is truly unique and something that only vet professionals will understand fully. But alas, I didn't; I sat there in my own self-pity and wallowed.

My mind kept going back to a meeting with my very first boss. I had been a vet for under a year and was trying to find my way, trying to be the best vet I possibly could. Something I struggled with was charging people the full amount for the care I provided. I couldn't see why I should charge the same amount of money for a consult as a senior vet would who had been in the game upwards of ten years. At the time, I had started shaving off costs here and there, not charging fees for dispensing medications, not charging my time for taking bloods from an animal, charging half a consult when it didn't take the full fifteen minutes. I saw it as my way of making myself value for money. My boss did not. I was called in for a meeting, sat down like a naughty school child and shown a list of all the times I had 'made allowances' or given away services for discounted prices. I tried to explain myself to my boss, telling her that I felt that it was unfair to the client that they got me for the same price as a senior vet.

'Do you know what your problem is, Rory?' she said, after listening to me stumble and rabbit on about not feeling as if I was good value for money. 'Your problem is you want everyone to like you.'

I stopped and thought about it. She was saying it as if that was a bad thing, like it was my downfall. 'So I shouldn't want people to like me?' I replied facetiously. I really couldn't understand what she meant. It was the way I had always been and I knew no differently.

'No, I don't mean that, I mean that the only reason you do the things you do, like give away cheap consults, is so the clients will like you.'

Again, I was confused. Surely if clients liked you they were going to come back to see you again? God forbid, you might have a good relationship with your clients! I was a bit taken aback by the exchange, but I accepted what she had said and promised to stop giving so many discounts.

Lying in bed that morning, I kept thinking back to the meeting, wondering if that was really my issue. Did I have some deep-seated issue that meant I needed everyone to like me? Was I a broken human being? And if so, why? I had had a normal upbringing. I was from a wonderful, loving family. I lay there for hours, eventually getting out of bed at two in the afternoon. That was so unlike me; I am, and always have been, an early riser. I went into the living room and put the TV on, some rubbish American sit-com. I made a cuppa and went to get my phone. I had loads of missed calls from work and texts from one of the receptionists and my boss. The text from the receptionist read, 'Rory, the Kims are here; they need to speak to you – call me if you can.' I have never been able to stay away from work on my days off and immediately dialled the work number.

'Hey Rory, don't worry, I think it's okay for now. They were just in earlier and they didn't know what to do – they wanted to talk to you and get some advice.'

'Okay, I'll speak to them tomorrow. I'm not really sure how I can help – I'm hardly an expert in the legalities of cat ownership.' (There's another job title you can add to the list of veterinary sub-specialties.)

'Oh, hang on, before you go, hold on.' The phone went quiet and then onto hold music: she was transferring the call.

My boss picked up the phone. 'Hi Rory, have you seen my text?'

'Oh no, I'm sorry – I saw you had messaged but didn't read it before calling in. All okay?'

'Yes, fine, I just need you to write me an account of your consult yesterday, the one where you got the cat signed over. The owner has called in saying he is not happy and feels you forced him to do something he didn't want to do.'

I could have screamed. 'You're joking!' I half shouted down the phone.

'No, I'm afraid not. He has written in a formal complaint and I just need your side of the story. Don't worry, I'm sure it will be fine, we just need to go through the process. If you could write an account of what happened and email it to me I can discuss with him later on. Is that okay?'

I had almost stopped listening, I was full of anger and hatred and wanted to throw something. 'Yes, okay,' I snapped, 'I'll email it later, bye.' I hung up.

'Could this week get any worse?' I thought, punching a pillow on my sofa in anger. How can I be in trouble for trying to do another thing right? It just didn't seem fair. I chucked on an old pair of jeans, a T-shirt and a baseball cap and grabbed my laptop. I stomped my way to the pub, which was three doors down from my flat. I ordered a pint of Guinness and sat and wrote my account. Once I had finished, I ordered another pint and then re-read it. I had to rewrite most of it. It wasn't rude, but I had used some rather fruity language in expressing my frustration at the situation. I had even signed off with '. . . and that is why, in my opinion, some people should just not be allowed to own a pet. Yours sincerely, Dr Rory Cowlam BVetMed PGCertSurg (WBIS) MRCVS'. The post-nominals were wanky but I left them to make a point.

I sent the email to my boss, the edited version, and sat back with my third pint. I thought writing the email would make me feel better, help me get rid of some of my anger, but if anything I felt worse. The only thing that had helped at all with my mood was the black nectar sat in my right hand. I knew it was the wrong way to approach it but self-medication with alcohol seemed to be my preferred coping strategy that day, so I sat in the pub for the rest of the afternoon. I bought some fried chicken on my way home and collapsed into bed in a drunken stupor.

*

Friday. Ouch. My head was banging and as I woke up to my shrill alarm I immediately regretted not drinking water before bed. The fried chicken from the night before was on my bedroom floor and had given the room a lovely aroma. I stumbled to the bathroom, looked in the mirror, and hardly recognised the person looking back at me. Coffee, water, paracetamol was my morning routine and I drove into work, trying not to do the maths in my head to work out if I was still over the limit.

I slunk into work and made another coffee before busying myself by catching up on notes and emails from the day before. I hadn't heard the latest from the Kims or whether my boss had managed to handle the complaint from Scratchy's owner, but I didn't really want to think about either at that point. Scratchy, the flea-ridden cat, was still at work, so I went into the cat ward to give him a cuddle. He was really sweet and maybe it was wishful thinking, but I was sure his skin was looking happier. I shouted to the nurse on with me that morning; I wanted to take some bloods to make sure Scratchy was well and I hadn't missed something. After all, if this was going to be a complaint, I wanted to prove that he was healthy and I was right.

I picked him and gave him a cuddle, walking through to prep. The nurse was waiting. She was a student nurse called Tessa, really sweet and eager to learn. When vet nurses train, they spend a lot of time in practice, essentially learning on the job, a bit like vet students.

Tessa had set everything up, a needle and syringe, a spirit swab to disinfect the skin before taking the blood and some clippers to remove the hair from Scratchy's neck. I gave her the cat and thanked her for setting up. She held Scratchy while I carefully clipped the hair and cleaned the skin, and then I popped the needle through the surface and tried to draw back on his jugular vein. No blood came so I repositioned my syringe, pushing slightly deeper into the cat's neck. As I repositioned, Scratchy decided this was not his favourite thing to be doing on a Friday morning and made a bid for freedom. Holding cats for bloods is an art form, and one that takes years of practice. Without a good nurse holding the cat for blood taking, you will never get the bloods, period. Unfortunately, despite Tessa being a very accomplished student, holding cats was simply not her forte. Cats are wonderful creatures – they can sense what you're feeling before you're even aware of it, so often if you're not one hundred percent confident when holding a cat, they will know, and foil you in an instant.

Scratchy leapt upwards out of Tessa's arms, my needle and syringe flicking across the room in the process. I grabbed for the cat and held him tightly to me as he sunk his claws into my arm. I let him settle and checked his neck, which was fine. I put the cat back in his kennel. I was deathly silent and clenching my jaw so hard it was aching. I could feel a fire building inside me like I wanted to punch something, and as I picked up my needle and syringe I threw it as hard as I could at the wall. I dropped to my haunches, my head in my hands. What was wrong with me? It's not uncommon to have to try a few times to get blood from a cat, especially a wriggly one, but today I had no patience. I apologised to Tessa, who looked petrified, clearly not understanding my outburst, and I took myself off to my consult room.

I couldn't get Tessa's face out of my head – she had looked so frightened. It was at that moment I realised I had to do something about my behaviour. I had heard horror stories of old school vets who were rough with animals and lost their temper, not caring for their colleagues or patients. I was not going this way. If that was to be me, I was going to leave the profession.

I went to see my boss that day and discussed what I was feeling. I didn't know what it was but I was angry and upset and felt hard done by. I told her I needed a few days off and she very kindly obliged. This was not something that a lot of veterinary bosses would do at such short notice, but I think she could see I was hurting. I was scared that if I continued to work I was going to explode. I'm not sure my boss entirely knew how to handle the situation. She was clearly worried about my mental health but, at the same time, I think it surprised her as it seemed to come from nowhere. I don't know how others make it known when they are struggling;

from the research I have done it seems that most men suffer in silence. I certainly tried to. I'm sure I dropped some hints along the way, but probably only the kind of hints that close friends or family would have picked up on. I hadn't spoken to any of my close mates or family properly for a few weeks so they didn't know the extent of what I was dealing with. Not that I really did either. For the rest of the day I lay low, in my consult room just getting on with the job – thankfully it was mainly routine consults. I went home that evening with a plan: I was going to get therapy, and that was that.

10

The End of the Road

Everyone always asks what it's like to euthanise an animal, often commenting that it must be such a hard thing to do and wondering how I cope with it. I think I shock a lot of people when I tell them that actually it's often not the worst part of the job. Yes, it's hugely emotional and difficult to end an animal's life, but I am a firm believer that we as vets are incredibly lucky to have euthanasia as a valid and fair option for our patients, and also our clients. Whenever I discuss euthanasia in animals, I am always interested to hear people's opinion. Should we be allowed to do it? Is it the right thing to do? Is it an abuse of human power? I know where my opinion lies but it is a very interesting discussion to have.

What I find even more relevant and intriguing is the extension of that conversation to human euthanasia and whether it should be allowed. Clearly this is a contested topic, with some people viewing it as a practice of murder, while others see it as a way of ending suffering in terminally ill patients. As a veterinarian who deals with death and euthanasia on a regular basis, I cannot help but think that euthanasia should be a practice in human medicine. Yes, it would have to be tightly regulated, and yes, you would need more than a single doctor's opinion. In fact, you would probably need to put the decision to a court of doctors to make sure it was the majority decision, but I believe that if we could find a way of incorporating this into the healthcare service, huge amounts of suffering and pain could be avoided. I am hugely lucky to have a healthy family and I have only lost one grandmother, and that was relatively sudden and quick. I cannot begin to imagine the pain of terminal disease, when you know nothing can cure you and all you want is to die. Surely introducing euthanasia for these cases is the only right and just thing to do? Thankfully, this is not something for me to decide, but all I know is that I am truly grateful that we in the veterinary profession have euthanasia as an option, as it is often the fairest and most ethical choice.

As a vet I have euthanised many animals, and as a pet owner I have had to have more than a dozen pets put to sleep. I think to truly understand the emotional toll of losing an animal, you have to go through it yourself. I lost my first pet, Creamy the cat, when I was in my early teens. I was there – I saw her lifeless body. It was utterly heart-breaking but it makes me a better vet today. Having some understanding of what the sobbing client in front of you is going through can help them feel more comfortable, even if it is only a tiny, tiny bit.

There were two pieces of advice that Mr Benson, our vet, gave to me and my family when we had to go through this process. Number one, if you think it's time, then list your pet's five favourite things to do, whether that's chase a ball, sleep in front of the fire, cuddle up on the sofa, scoff down their dinner or chase the cat. If they aren't doing some of these things then it's likely their quality of life is starting to take a turn. Once they're down to only doing two or three of those five, it's probably time. Number two, and this is something that I couldn't agree more with, is that you are better to make the decision to put your pet to sleep a week too early than a day too late. There is nothing I hate more than getting a call from an owner who says their pet has been struggling for weeks, weeing and pooing all over the house and hardly able to get around. As a loving owner, it is completely understandable to want to hang on until the very last moment, but often it is far beyond when the animal starts to suffer.

I think it is important that, as a pet owner, you have an open dialogue about these things with your vet, who is there to offer guidance and support. By no means am I saying you should do everything your vet says and euthanise your pet on the spot if they suggest it, but often together you can make sure it is the right time. You, and only you, know your pet best, so never let someone question your judgement, but often a vet can pick up pain and other signs of discomfort earlier than your animal will let on. Whether it's planned weeks in advance, at your house, with the family around, or whether it's an emergency bloody mess and you're having to make a snap decision, it's never easy.

*

There is one particular euthanasia that has stuck with me over the last few years and it started on one particular winter's morning. A call came in about ten o'clock – it was an elderly dog, unable to stand on its back legs, struggling. The owner was told to come straight in (we always accommodate these cases as soon as we can) and I assessed the dog – Rupert. He had the grizzled muzzle of an older soul, with kind eyes and a submissive nature. You could tell from a mile off that he wasn't right. He had managed to stand and stumble into the clinic, but only just, swaying in like a drunk cowboy. He was weak and clearly feeling very woolly, and at the age of sixteen, this was a worry. I took a look over him and found nothing obvious other than a low-ish temperature and some mild discomfort in his abdomen. There was no sign of an abdominal tumour, his heart sounded fine and his circulation, though he was dehydrated, seemed okay. I recommended that we do some blood work to get a better idea of what was going on – it's hard to assess how serious these things are without testing. Rupert just lay there on his side as we clipped and prepped his jugular vein, and carefully removed 3ml of dark red blood. I was beginning to get quite concerned at how compliant he was being and when his blood presented itself into my syringe it was dark, darker than was normal. He was definitely dehydrated, but there was something else going on here. I had this really strong feeling. Fifteen minutes later we started to get some results trickle through onto my lab monitor and it was not good. This wonderful old dog's kidneys had packed in and unfortunately it looked like there was no way he was going to make a decent recovery. His only chance was some pretty intensive care over the next few days, and even that had no guarantees.

I called the client and discussed next steps and options. We decided to give him the day to see if we could get him to perk up at all or start eating, which he hadn't done in almost five days. My nurse and I placed an intravenous catheter into Rupert and started fluid therapy. Often the only real approach to kidney disease is to put the animal on a high rate of fluids to try to rehydrate them and flush out all the toxins that have built up in their blood stream. I also gave him some decent pain relief and an anti-nausea injection to make him feel better and, hopefully, start him eating something. I spent most of the day either sitting with Rupert, trying to coax him into eating and offering him comfort, or on the phone to his owner giving regular updates. By mid-afternoon it was becoming pretty clear that we weren't going to get a miraculous recovery. I called the owner for the final time that day and suggested the family come into the clinic to discuss what we would do. If at all possible I try to have these final conversations in person: it's much easier to gauge emotion when you're face-to-face with someone. The owner agreed and asked if she could wait another hour to pick up her children from school so they could come with her. I knew at that point she understood what had to happen. 'Of course, that's fine,' I said calmly down the phone – after all, who am I to deprive her children of a last goodbye to their pet?

The minutes dragged by as four o'clock approached. I spent the last half an hour setting up my consult room as some sort of morbid hospital room for the lovely old dog. He was sprawled out on his side on a vet bed (one of those really comfy-looking, thick mats) on top of an 8in thick mattress. His drip line ran from his front leg and I managed to hook the fluid bag onto the window fixing. If he had been feeling better he would have definitely walked around and pulled his intravenous catheter out but this little guy was going nowhere: all he wanted to do was sleep. I was sitting with him, gently stroking him on the head when I heard the front door of the clinic 'bing'. I slowly got to my feet and poked my head round the consult room door: the whole family was there. I nodded at them and beckoned them into the room. Tentatively they trudged through the door and as soon as they saw their dog they all collapsed to the floor around him, showering him with tears, kisses and love. I gave them five minutes to reacquaint themselves with him, and then addressed the matter at hand. I looked at the mother and then at the children – they couldn't have been older than five and seven. I gave the mother a knowing look and she just raised her hand. 'We have come to a decision,' she said, trying to project an air of calm and authority, but I could see straight through it, and knew she was just putting it on for the kids.

I let the family take as long as they wanted saying goodbye to their dog of thirteen years. I spent most of the time making myself busy in the prep room – cleaning, tidying, moving things from one place to another and then back again. After about ten minutes I popped my head around the door and from what I could gather in that hugely emotional moment, the family were gearing up to leave. I have come to learn over the years that no two euthanasias are the same. One main difference between owners is that some stay with their pets while they pass away and some opt not to. In this case it was the latter. I entered the room and the mother looked at me, her mascara now forming black runways down her cheeks. She looked away and said to the father, 'Come on, let's go.'

Until this point I hadn't really interacted with the man of the family. He was quite large and clearly trying to hold it together for his family. It's odd in my job, you deal with the extremes of emotion: utter sadness, sheer aggression, huge disappointment and unadulterated elation. In my experience, though, it's always the big guys that take the sad times the hardest. I don't know whether it's because they try so hard to hide it, but there is something devastating in seeing a 6ft-something behemoth of a man give in to the tears and bawl over his ill pet. In this case he did manage to hold back the tears and put an arm around his wife, gave me a nod and ushered the children away from the motionless dog.

The daughter dutifully followed with one final kiss to her first-ever pet but the son stayed standing where he had been since entering the room. I had hardly noticed in the intensity of that room, but the youngest member of the family had barely moved, spoken or shown any emotion since entering. He had walked in behind his towering father, stood in the corner and just taken in the whole experience like a statue.

A question I'm asked a lot is whether it's right for children to see and experience this side of pet ownership. I am a firm believer that it's an important (and hard) lesson for children to learn, and parents generally know best how their kids will cope with it, but I think, if at all possible, children should be taught about the 'circle of life' from a young age. This particular experience, though, definitely made me think twice about my stance. As I stood looking at the ashen face of the young lad, it seemed as if he couldn't quite compute what was happening. When he had got up that morning, he had left for school as normal, leaving his four-legged pal in its bed at home. Now here he was, in an odd clinical room with Rupert laying on a vet's bed, and he was being told he had to leave him. The father came back into the room and called to him, 'Come on Peter, it's time to go.' The little boy walked over to his dog and stood there looking at him. I remember trying to work out what he was thinking. Every day since he was born, he had woken up in a house of his mum, his dad, his sister and his dog. As of tomorrow, this wouldn't be the case anymore. I remember resisting every urge to go over and kneel down beside him to try to console him. I just watched. He knelt down next to the dog's head and paused. What happened next will forever stay with me and even now, as I think about it, I well up. Have you ever seen a person's heart break? Well, I am convinced that I did that day. The boy was on his knees next to his best friend and it was as if every part of that last half hour hit him at once. His body convulsed as he fell onto the dog and let out a wail that could have risen the dead. His father took a step into the room and scooped up his limp form as he carried on crying. They left, closing the door behind them, and I sat there trying to comprehend what I had witnessed, tears falling from my chin.

Almost on autopilot I got up, gathered the injection and attached it to Rupert's intravenous catheter. As I pushed the plunger of the syringe, I stroked him and told him how loved he was. He slipped away peacefully and I stayed with him for what felt like an hour, my head hanging between my knees, tears pooling on the floor. One of the nurses came in and found me and threw a hug around me as I got up off the floor. The receptionist made me a cup of tea and we sat together in silence for a few minutes. It's times like this that I really love, and I mean love, our profession and the people I work with. No-one said anything, we sat drinking our tea, silently consoling and supporting each other.

Just like that it was back to work. Fifteen minutes after one of the most harrowing euthanasias I have ever done and I was back smiling at another client, talking about what to feed her new kitten, no trace of Rupert or his family, just a faint lingering hint of air freshener the only clue that something not-so-nice may have happened in the not-so-distant past. One thing that has become abundantly clear to me over the last five years is that there is no part of this job that is normal. The seesawing from happy-go-lucky with a client and their healthy, happy pet, to being plunged into an intensely emotional situation such as that with Rupert, and then straight back to easygoing again happens every day in veterinary practices all around the country.

*

Euthanising any animal can be gut-wrenchingly emotional, just like Rupert, but even that can't compare to losing an animal of your own. Thankfully it has been a few years since I last said goodbye to one of my family's dogs but I remember it like it was yesterday. I was working on a Saturday at one of the branch practices of my first job. I was the only vet there and on the front desk was Gill, one of the receptionists. She was mid-thirties, blonde, with clear blue eyes. We had got on well from day one. I had been warned that she could be a touch 'stand-off-ish' by one of the other receptionists when I had started but we never had an issue. She was a mum of two and, even though she was only ten to fifteen years older than I was, she looked out for me. She would supply me with cups of tea aplenty and book me off ten minutes on the diary for a break, making sure I ate regularly through the day. Better than that, though, she gave the best hugs. I had always been a bit of a 'mummy's boy' and being a hundred miles from my family was something I really struggled with, so I always welcomed her thoughtfulness.

We were having a coffee and a catch-up. I had just finished some of my morning consults and hit one of Gill's breaks. We were chatting about our weekend. The Saturday shift was annoying, part of the job, but it finished at three in the afternoon so there was plenty of the weekend left to enjoy. Gill was telling me about her plans to take her dogs to the beach when my phone buzzed in my pocket. I looked down at the caller ID to see the name 'Dad' flashing on the screen of my iPhone. I excused myself from Gill and answered the call with mild apprehension – my dad knew I was working and he wouldn't call usually.

'Dad? All okay?' I answered, sensing something was wrong.

'Yeah, not too bad,' he lied.

'What's wrong?' My parents have never been able to lie to me.

'Poppy isn't great,' he said. Poppy was our Great Dane at the time. We got her when I was about sixteen and she had been there through my veterinary training. She was the most ridiculous dog. Wonderfully stupid and incredibly loving. She loved nothing better than doing the 'Great Dane lean' as our family had termed it. All you big breed dog owners out there will know what I mean. Dogs of a certain size develop this habit of coming up beside you and leaning their entire weight into you, as if they can't be bothered to hold themselves up and expect you to do it for them. I regularly found myself on the floor having been pushed over by Poppy or, alternatively, pinned against the wall. Being a Great Dane, she was a weighty dog. Unfortunately, not long after I qualified as a vet, she had been diagnosed with heart disease. This is something that Great Danes are a bit prone to. The disease in particular is dilated cardiomyopathy, commonly known as DCM. Poppy's heart had been getting progressively bigger and bigger, stretching like a balloon being inflated. This, as you can probably guess, is not ideal, and she had recently gone into full blown heart failure. I had been trying to manage her as a case from London, while my parents were back in the Cotswolds with the help of Mr Benson (remember him?).

This is one thing I'm not sure I was prepared for after university. My parents had spent a huge amount of money putting me through school and veterinary school and now they could ask my opinion on our family's pets. It wasn't just my parents either – suddenly I was inundated with messages from friends asking my opinion and advice on their animals. I like to think it's because they valued my opinion, but I think more often than not it was just to avoid a veterinary bill. Slightly frustratingly for both me and them, though, there is only so much I can do from a history and a photo. Without access to the animal for an exam, diagnostics or medications, asking me is about as useful as asking any Tom, Dick or Harry. I have already mentioned my deep-seated need to help people, especially people I care about, and this sudden influx of questions didn't half bring a mound of pressure with it. Every part of my being wants to help anyone who needs me, but more often than not I find myself replying to messages with the words, 'Go to your vet.'

With my parents though, it was difficult. I was a new vet and Poppy was a pretty complicated case. Not only had she gone into heart failure but she had also developed a condition called atrial fibrillation. If you remember your GCSE biology, you will recall that the top two chambers of the heart are called the atria. Atrial fibrillation is when these two chambers decide for whatever reason that they no longer want to beat and pump blood into the bottom chambers (ventricles for you biology nerds), so instead they sort of flutter and vibrate. This is not very efficient and often leads to issues, like with Poppy. The sentence 'Poppy isn't great' could have meant many things. My dad went on to explain that it in fact meant that Poppy was lying on the floor, unable to get up with a belly full of fluid.

'She's a bit fucked then, Dad,' I said, trying to lighten the mood.

'Yup, I think she is. We're going to call Rod out today,' he replied. I knew exactly what that meant.

'I'm on my way – don't you dare do it until I'm home,' I said and hung up the phone as tears started to well up in my eyes.

*

I'm not sure how normal jobs work. Do they give compassionate leave for the loss of a pet? If not, they bloody well should. Honestly, I wasn't sure what our company policy was on that day but I sure as hell knew I wasn't sticking around to ask. I had two hours left of my shift but there was no way I could concentrate now, and I most definitely was not spending the next few hours vaccinating a few animals while my dog was lying at death's door back home in the Cotswolds. I walked back through the practice to the front desk. Gill heard me coming and looked up from the computer screen. She immediately knew something wasn't right, possibly due to my panicked walk, more likely due to my bloodshot eyes.

'My dog is dying – I have to go,' I blurted out, emotion removing any sort of coherent thought from my mind.

'I'll sort everything. Go!' she said, throwing her arms round me for the biggest hug I had ever received. The hug gave me strength and I left, got in my car and drove. It was early afternoon on a Saturday so there was little traffic. I got onto the M4 and sat there in the outside lane, overtaking car after car. I couldn't help myself picturing Poppy. Every part of me yearned to be by her side. All I hoped was that she was comfortable and I wasn't making my parents hold on while she was lying there suffering. I had visions of her lying flat out on her side struggling to breathe. I got to Junction 16 and pulled off the motorway. I flew down the country lanes and pulled up at Manor Cottage, my childhood home. I clocked the time as I switched off the engine: one hour and fifty minutes. A new record.

I burst in through the utility door and walked through the house to find Poppy and my parents all sitting on the floor in the sitting room. My mum was holding a bowl of water to Poppy's mouth for her to lap (one of the side effects of heart disease medication is you get very thirsty and need to drink a lot, especially when you're a Great Dane). I knelt down at Poppy's side and gave her a kiss, and her tail thumped into the floor. She had slobber dripping down from her jowls so I wiped them with my jumper sleeve. I have always regarded my pets as part of the family. I'm not sure that non-dog people understand. I wouldn't ever think twice about wiping the slobber from our dog's mouths or giving them a lick of my ice cream.

Poppy had been there for me through a lot of hard times. Whenever I had come home from university she had been there. We had spent countless evenings cuddling on the floor watching TV and covered thousands of miles over the fields around our home. The vet was on his way out to our house so my parents and I made a cup of tea and sat with our dog of eight years. Before the vet arrived, my dad had to leave. He had a work trip. I got up to say goodbye to him and gave him a hug. I don't recall seeing my dad cry over as a kid. My earliest recollection of him in tears is in fact when I was fourteen. One of his closest friends passed away. Before that I can't actually remember seeing him upset. As I hugged him though, I felt him start to go, and, sure enough, as we said goodbye, his eyes were bloodshot and his face was screwed up with emotion. I have always struggled seeing grown men cry. I don't know exactly why, perhaps because even now men's vulnerability is still so hidden away. Seeing my dad cry, though – that's a whole next level.

My mum and I sat with Poppy until we heard the sound of tyres on gravel outside. Poppy just lay there. Ordinarily she would have been up at the door barking to warn off the intruders. A Great Dane bark is a scary thing but Poppy was always all bark, no bite. As soon as you gave her a bit of fuss or sat down, she was your best mate. The vet came in and placed his kit on the floor next to Poppy.

It wasn't Mr Benson, our vet for the last twenty years. It was his junior partner, Mr Babb. He was a big guy, easily over 6ft and built like a rugby player. He did the majority of the farm work at the practice but he had an incredibly soft manner. I had once seen him come in from a farm visit, see some puppies waiting in reception and get on the floor to roll around with them. He was a lovely guy, and he treated Poppy with the same gentle manner I had seen time and time again whilst shadowing him as a vet student. I watched as Mr Babb prepared a tourniquet and the injection of euthatal that was about to put Poppy out of her suffering. I had a sudden realisation that I was the client in this situation, but I was caught between feeling my own grief and consoling my mum. I wasn't really sure what I should be doing in the situation so I just held my mum's hand and stroked Poppy's head.

Just like that, she was gone. I started sobbing. I had managed to hold it in mostly until that point but it all became too much all at once. I looked at Mr Babb and apologised, mumbling something about being silly and I should know better. He looked at me with a knowing look as my body shook while I tried to hold in the sobs. I reached down and put my forehead to Poppy's like I had always done, as if to tell her a secret. My tears rolled onto her motionless face and I gave her a final kiss.

Mr Babb put his hand on my shoulder and asked if I was okay.

'Yup, I'll be fine,' I replied, 'It's always so bloody hard when it's your own.' I trailed off as I wiped the tears away on my shirt sleeve.

'It never gets easier,' he said, truthfully.

I gave him a hand carrying Poppy to the car. She was almost 60kg and it was no mean feat at all. Carrying any dead animal is an art form, to be fair. It has its booby traps. When you euthanise an animal, everything relaxes. All muscle tone that there once was disappears, and this means quite often there is a bit of leakage. It is not uncommon then for a euthanised animal to urinate and/or defecate (definitely pass wind), and quite often these animals are rather ill, meaning their movements are rather disgusting. Poppy managed to hold it all in thankfully. Not that I would have really minded, of course. We placed her in the back of Mr Babb's pick-up and I gave her one last kiss. Then my mum and I stood with our arms around each other as the vet drove away with our beloved dog.

*

I went back to work on the Monday and was immediately called to my bosses' office. Here it was, the reprimand for leaving early that I had been expecting. I walked in, building my defence in my head as I went. My boss, a short, sharp-featured woman with a greyish-blonde bob, put a hand on my arm as I headed past her to the chair and gave me a hug. I wasn't entirely sure she was capable of human emotion but she was hugging me (weird). I was shell-shocked and sat down a bit bemused. 'Are you okay, Rory? I heard about the weekend,' she said, with what I identified as empathy in her voice.

'Um, yes I'm okay. Sorry for . . .' I started.

'Nonsense, it's fine – I completely understand.' She cut me off. 'Blimey,' I thought to myself, 'had I got away with it?'

'I just wanted to make sure you're okay,' she said. And just like that, I thanked her and turned to leave. As I reached the door, she coughed. 'Ah, and I'll take the two hours out of your pay.' So close, and yet so far.

The whole team was lovely. When you work with animal people, they just 'get it'. No explanations needed, hugs offered in dozens and Rose even bought me lunch to make sure I was okay. It was like a relative had died, and, to animal people, when a pet dies it really is like losing a relative.

*

If I look back at my own animals that I have lost or had to say goodbye to, I remember things that vets have said to me or things they have done which made the process easier. I think it's something a lot of vets will do over their careers: they try to find the recipe for the best possible euthanasia. I almost found it once, but it was so special, I worry I may never be able to replicate it.

I came in one morning and sat in front of the computer. I looked at the diary and my heart sunk slightly as I saw a home euthanasia appointment booked in for later in the day. Daisy had been coming to the practice since it opened back in 2013. She was a little cairn terrier with buckets of attitude. She used to tolerate me but, as time went on, she became less and less amenable in the clinic. I never held it against her and often found myself chuckling, telling her it was okay as she tried to bite at the air around my hands and arms. Despite her nature, I had a real soft spot for Daisy as she had become a bit of a regular at the vet's over the last year or two. She had been diagnosed as diabetic and, despite our best efforts, had become quite ill over recent time. The final straw was that she had recently developed cataracts in both her eyes, leaving her as blind as a bat, and she really wasn't coping very well. I got on with her owner too – she was a lovely middle-aged lady called Mrs Fallows. Mrs F was very mild mannered and spent the majority of her appointments apologising for her dog's behaviour, much to my amusement.

'Oh please, Mrs F, you have to stop apologising – she is just trying to give me a love bite,' I used to laugh as Daisy tried to take my fingers off.

Aggressive dogs are something most vets deal with on a semi-regular basis. Some are a real issue but Daisy never posed much of a problem, and to this day I genuinely don't think she ever meant to hurt me. I wasn't surprised when I saw she was booked in and I wrote my name against the appointment to make sure I was the one to see her. I jumped in the car with veterinary nurse 'G' just after lunch. G was a bit of a legend. She was young and swore like a trooper, but she was one of the best nurses I had ever worked with. Behind closed doors, if she was comfortable with you, G would crack jokes, dirty as you like. She was an awesome person to work with and we got on really well, often competing to make the same joke before the other. The great thing about G, though, was her ability to turn from morale-boosting joker into serious super nurse in a matter of seconds. It is people like G that make the veterinary profession so bloody amazing.

We drove to Mrs F's house and parked on the cobbled drive. 'Fuck me,' said G as we pulled up. The house was massive. I knocked the lion-head knocker on the huge front door and Mrs F pulled the door open for us. She was only a small woman and I was quite impressed at how easily she manoeuvred the gigantic wooden door.

'Hi Rory, come on in,' she said, ushering us into the entrance hall. 'Go on through to the kitchen; you'll find her in there.'

We wandered through, taking in the incredible artwork on the walls, the sculpted wooden staircase and marble flooring as we went. The kitchen was, predictably, enormous, with a long oak table as the centrepiece. The whole kitchen was surrounded by floor to ceiling windows opening onto a perfectly kept garden. I was just thinking how I wanted to live somewhere like that when Daisy came up behind me and started sniffing at my shoes. The wonderful thing about blind dogs is they often remember their home and navigate via a mental map. I've seen blind dogs sidestep plant pots and manoeuvre around door frames with expert accuracy. They really are incredible animals. I leant down to Daisy and offered her my hand. This was the point that she would usually start backing away and telling me off, and I prepared myself to withdraw my hand at speed. She sniffed carefully and then, for the first time ever, followed it with a little lick. She pushed my hand with her nose to put my fingers on top of her head for a scratch. I sat down on the floor, gently tickling her behind the ears and she sat next to me. This had never happened before and I was so shocked that I hadn't clocked Mrs F's face of astonishment as she had followed us through to the kitchen.

'Wha ... What is she doing?' Mrs F said in wonder, as Daisy sat down next to me and curled up with my hand scratching her on the head.

'We have finally made friends, Mrs F,' I said, beaming up at her. It was perfect.

G drew up some sedation that would make Daisy so sleepy she wouldn't feel the catheter I was going to place in her leg. I stayed sitting next to Daisy and carried on dutifully making a fuss. If I tried to stop she would look around as if to say, 'Where is your bloody hand and why isn't it stroking me?' So needy. G handed me the syringe and I decided to risk it. I increased the vigour of my scratching with my left hand and with my right, jabbed in a sharp motion, popping the needle into Daisy's back leg. She didn't move. She only realised something was happening when I very slowly started to inject the sedation but a cursory glance was all I got. I almost had to pinch myself. This dog was usually untouchable but today she had sought me out, sat with me and just allowed me to inject her. I was gobsmacked. Mrs F had been watching on, glistening tears silently running down her cheeks.

'She knows,' she said, as I looked up at her.

'She does,' I replied.

Mrs F went to the cupboard and grabbed one of Daisy's favourite chews. As soon as the cupboard opened, Daisy was up and waiting, tail wagging. She almost had her owner's hand off in taking the chew – I don't know whether it was because she was blind or whether she was just terribly trained but I didn't comment. She plodded through the kitchen and walked up to one of the sliding doors. Mrs F went over and opened it – Daisy really was a princess. She walked into the garden, found a spot on the decking and lay down to start going to town on her favourite snack. As she did, we went out to join her, sitting around a metal garden table. The sun was setting over the tall trees at the end of the garden and I couldn't help but feel at peace. There was something rather magical about that afternoon: we were saying goodbye to a cheeky little dog but it felt completely calm. We sat chatting about Daisy, watching on as she chewed away happily. She fell asleep with the bone in her mouth.

*

There never has been and never will be a more perfect euthanasia for me. Daisy, the dog that ordinarily would have hated me touching her, let alone trying to do anything to her, had accepted me and had seemed to understand what we were there to do. I had known Daisy's owner for years, and sitting drinking a cup of tea and reminiscing about Daisy's adventures as a younger dog was truly special. Mrs F had decided that she wanted to bury Daisy in their beautiful garden, underneath her favourite tree. She used to lie there in the summer months in the shade and watch the world go by. Mrs F had told me she was worried about foxes finding Daisy if she buried her too shallow and, without hesitation, I offered to come back after work and help her bury Daisy. She beamed at me through her tear-filled eyes and gave me a hug.

I returned to the mansion house after my evening consults. Mrs F answered the door and thrust a glass of champagne into my hand. 'We have to toast little Daisy now, don't we?' she said. I smiled at her and walked through the entrance hall.

We buried Daisy in a deep hole under her favourite tree with her bed, her favourite toy and a few of her favourite treats. I usually try not to cry in front of clients but both Mrs F and I had tears falling from our cheeks as we placed her little body into the ground.

People always think putting an animal to sleep is the worst part of being a vet, and sometimes it really is terrible. But this will go down as one of the most magical things I have ever done in my job, and I look back at it with sheer joy. Euthanasia is sad, yes, but, like anything in the veterinary world, it can be truly amazing too.

11

And now . . .

From delivering a lamb in a barn in the Cotswolds to being a veterinary surgeon in South London, these are my stories. It's been four and a half years since I qualified as a vet and twenty-three years since I first walked into Mr Benson's veterinary surgery. As I write the final words of this book, Tripod is sat on my lap sleeping, over a year after being brought into the vet's. I am pleased to say I am in a healthy mental space and continue to love practicing veterinary.

I count myself incredibly lucky to have been able to follow my dreams to becoming a vet and have so many people to thank for helping me along the way. Being a vet is tough – I hope I have shown you that – but, by God, the good outweighs the bad. Being trusted with someone's pet is a privilege and an honour, and something I will never take for granted. The veterinary world is filled with the most amazing people: vets, nurses and all the veterinary staff. I hope that by reading this book you have been shown a glimpse behind the prep room door, and given an insight into the inner workings of both a veterinary surgery as well as a young vet's mind.

In my short time as a vet, I have learnt so much.

Firstly, that animals are the purest thing in the world. They bring unadulterated joy and sheer sadness when we have to say goodbye.

Secondly, that animal people are wonderful. I will forever be amazed at the lengths people go for their pets.

Thirdly, that mental health is something we need to speak about and be more aware of. The stigma must go, the conversation must start and continue. If I had been dealt a very slightly different hand, I know it might not have worked out so well for me. Therapy is something I never thought I would have to consider but it saved me. It saved my passion and kept me practicing the thing that I love. This is absolutely not a veterinary-specific topic, not by any means. Experiences like mine, as mild as they may seem, need to be the fuel to start a change. I hope to see more support from all professions for their new members coming out of university. It is happening – changes are being made – but we can do more. We cannot keep seeing incredible, compassionate, empathetic, smart, amazing humans leave the veterinary profession because they haven't had the support network they needed.

And finally, the veterinary profession and the people in it are the best.

Full stop.

Acknowledgements

I owe so much to so many people. Firstly to Hannah, Becca and everyone at Hodder who have been amazing in welcoming me and supporting me through this process. To Carly for helping me produce a real-life book. Tom Wright, for believing in me so fiercely and being a true friend. Jonny, my agent, Katie, Stef and the rest of the awesome team at Crown. All my friends and teachers at the Royal Veterinary College, which is a family, not just a university.

To the people who helped me on my way to realising my childhood dream of becoming a vet: Alf Wight, Rod Benson, Serena Stevens and (the majority of) my school teachers. I owe you more than I can repay.

Of course, to Bethan for being the best sister I could ask for, my mum for always helping me and believing in me, my dad for setting me the best possible example of being a man.

And finally Rhianna, for being my closest advisor, my proofreader, for putting up with my procrastination, my mood swings, for supporting me and for becoming the guardian of my mental health. I love you.

Oh, and Rufus and Ben.